THE HEALTH OF NATIONS

KV-513-194

The Health of Nations

Medicine, disease and development in the Third World

Edited by
B. FOLASADE IYUN
YOLA VERHASSELT
J. ANTHONY HELLEN

Avebury

Aldershot • Brookfield USA • Hong Kong • Singapore • Sydney

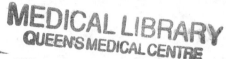

© B. F. Iyun, Y. Verhasselt and J. A. Hellen 1995

All rights reserved. No part of this publication may be reproduced, stored in a retrieval system, or transmitted in any form or by any means, electronic, mechanical, photocopying, recording or otherwise without the prior permission of the publisher.

Published by
Avebury
Ashgate Publishing Limited
Gower House
Croft Road
Aldershot
Hants GU11 3HR
England

Ashgate Publishing Company
Old Post Road
Brookfield
Vermont 05036
USA

British Library Cataloguing in Publication Data
Health of Nations: Disease, Medicine and
Development in the Third World
     I. Iyun, B. Folasade
     614.422724
ISBN   1 85628 922 2

Library of Congress Cataloging-in-Publication Data
Health of Nations: Disease, medicine and development
     in the Third World / edited by B. Folasade Iyun, Yola Verhasselt, Anthony J. Hellen
         p.   cm. Includes index.
     ISBN 1 85628 922 2 : £37.50 $67.95 (approx.)
1. Public health - Developing countries - Congresses.
   2. Environmental health - Developing countries - Congresses.
   3. Medical care - Developing countries - Congresses. I. Iyun, B. Folasade
   II. Verhasselt, Yola. III. Hellen, Anthony
   [DNLM : 1 World Health - Congresses. 2. Developing countries -
   Congresses. WA540 H236 1995]
RA441.5.H4545 1995   94-3754
614.4'09172'4--dc20   CIP

Reprinted 1996

Typeset by VIC Business & Computer Services Ltd
75 Agbowo Shopping Complex
Ibadan, Nigeria
Printed and bound by Athenaeum Press Ltd.,
Gateshead, Tyne & Wear

i001067395

Contents

List of figures

List of tables

List of contributors

A. K. Abiose
Department of Clinical Pharmacology
College of Medicine
Lagos University Teaching Hospital
Idi Araba, Lagos
Nigeria

O. Abosede
Institute of Child Health and Primary
  Health Care
College of Medicine
University of Lagos,
Idi-Araba, Lagos
Nigeria

Tunde Agbola
Centre for Urban and Regional Planning
Faculty of the Social Sciences
University of Ibadan
Ibadan, Nigeria

Rais Akhtar
Department of Geography
University of Kashmir
Srinagar J and K
India

O. A. Akinbamijo
Urban and Regional Planning Dept
Federal University of Technology
Akure, Ondo State
Nigeria

O.O. Akinkugbe
College of Medicine
University of Ibadan
Ibadan, Nigeria

Olabode Alokan
Department of Geography
University of Ibadan
Ibadan, Nigeria.

Juan, J. Burgos,
Centre of Biometeorological Research
National Council of Science and
Technology
Serrano 665
Buenos aires,
Argentina

Rodolfo, U. Carcavallo,
Institute of Zoonosis
Buenos Aires
Argentina

Susana Curto de Casas
Rivadavia 1653 1^0 B,
103 Buenos Aires,
Argentina

Daniel Dory
Department of Geography
University of Clermont - Ferrand
France

Layi Egunjobi
Centre for Urban and Regional Planning
University of Ibadan
Ibadan, Nigeria.

Adenike Emeke
Institute of Education
University of Ibadan,
Ibadan. Nigeria.

R. P. Gartoulla
Department of Clinical Pharmacology
Institute of Medicine
T.U. Teaching Hospital
P. O. B.x 3578
Kathmandu, Nepal
India

Peter Foggin
Universite de Montreal
Faculte des Arts et des Sciences
Department de Geographie
C.P. 6128 Succursale A
Montreal (Quebec) H3C 3 357
Canada

J. Anthony Hellen
Department of Geography
University of Newcastle-Upon-Tyne
Newcastle-Upon-Tyne NE1 7RU

U.A. Igun
Department of Sociology
University of Maiduguri
Maiduguri
Nigeria.

B. Folasade Iyun
Department of Geography
University of Ibadan
Ibadan, Nigeria

Tan Jian'an
Department of Chemical Geography
Institute of Geography
Chinese Academy of Sciences
P.O. Box 771, Building 917
Datun Road, Beijing, 100 - 101
China.

K.K. Kafle
Department of Clinical Pharmacology
Institute of Medicine
T.U. Teaching Hospital
P.O. Box 3578
Kathmandu, Nepal

T. Yu. Karimova
Department of Geography
Moscow State University
119899, Moscow
Russia

S. B. Karkee
Department of Clinical Pharmacology
Institute of Medicine
T.U. Teaching Hospital
P.O. Box 3578
Kathmandu, Nepal
India

Maria Los Angeles Y. Lopex
Institute of Zoonosis
Buenos Aires
Argentina

Richard Laing
Management Sciences for Health
165 Allandale Road
Boston, Massachusetts 02130
U.S.A.

A.F.B. Mabadeje
Department of Clinical Pharmacology
College of Medicine
Lagos University Teaching Hospital
Idi-Araba, Lagos
Nigeria.

Akin A. Mabogunje
Chairman,
Community Banks Commission
Abuja, Nigeria

Svetlana M. Malkhazova
Department of Geography
Moscow State University
119899, Moscow,
Russia.

Elizabeth Omoluabi
INED
27, rue du Commandeur
75675 Paris Cedex 14
France.

T. Ademola Oyejide
Department of Economics
University of Ibadan
Ibadan.
Nigeria

Y.M.S. Pradham
Department of Clinical Pharmacology
Institute of Medicine
T.U. Teaching Hospital
P.O.Box 3578
Kathmandu, Nepal
India

Li Ribang,
Institute of Geography
Chinese Academy of Sciences
Beijin 100101
China

Carlos Mena Segura
Institute of Zoonosis
Buenos Aires
Argentina

Hou Shaofan
Institute of Geography
Chinese Academy of Sciences
Beijin 100101

Dora J. Shehu
Department of Geography
Usman Dan Fodio University
Sokoto,
Nigeria

A. D. Shresth
Department of Clinical Pharmacology
Institute of Medicine
T. U. Teaching Hospital
P. O. Box 3578

Kathmandu, Nepal
India

Adedoyin Soyibo
Department of Economics
University of Ibadan
Ibadan.
Nigeria

Elizabeth Thomas-Hope
Department of Geography
Roxby Building
The University of Liverpool
P.O. Box 147
Liverpool L 69 3BX
U.K.

Bola Udegbe
Department of Psychology
Faculty of the Social Sciences
University of Ibadan
Ibadan, Nigeria.

Y.A.D.S. Wanasinghe
Department of Geography
University of Sri Jayewardenepura
Gangodawila, Nugegoda
Sri Lanka

Zhu Wenya,
Institute of Geography
Chinese Academy of Sciences
Beijin 100101
China

Wang Wuyi,
Institute of Geography
Chinese Academy of Sciences
Beijin 100101
China

T. W. Yoloye
Institute of Education
University of Ibadan
Ibadan.Nigeria

Preface

The conference on Health Issues in Development of which the book is the outcome was organized at the University of Ibadan by Dr. B. Folasade Iyun under the auspices of the Commission on Health and Development of the International Geographical Union. We are indebted to the University of Ibadan for the hospitality. Sixty-six participants belonging to 20 countries attended the conference. Thirty seven papers were presented. A selection is published in this volume. A broad range of topics was covered. The papers are grouped into five sections corresponding to main themes of the geographical approach of health and development.

Environmental changes are one of the main health hazards occurring in developing countries. In the first section of the book, several aspects of health consequences of environmental changes are examined, such as the consequences of global climate change which would affect the distribution of tropical diseases. The problem of increasing agricultural production responding to the needs of a fast growing population is particularly acute in Africa. Its environmental consequences upon endemic diseases have been modelled and mapped. An example of a positive effect of rural development upon health is demonstrated in China (with the decline of endemic disease incidence in selenium deficit areas). The overwhelming problem of clean water supply in developing countries is illustrated by the case of guinea worm diffusion in West Africa.

Rapid urbanization is a major challenge, also for health. Housing conditions, sanitation, environmental problems constitute health hazards in many fast growing cities of the developing world. As a result, malnutrition, infectious and parasitic diseases are still high in the poor urban areas. Several examples are detailed in the second section of this book. Moreover, the epidemiologic transition diffuse from the big cities. Westernization of diet and life style initiate the increase of chronic diseases (cardiovascular and cancers). The consequences of changing life styles are the theme of the third section. Various aspects are examined: the increase of cardiovascular diseases in Nigeria, geopsychiatric problems in the developing world, the changing health status in two traditional populations and the impact of tourism upon health. The particular relationship of women and health is approached in the fourth section.

The overwhelming importance of education and the role of women upon health need to be stressed. These features are analysed in the book: child health and its seasonal fluctuation, women and agricultural development and the problem of ageing.

Health care provision is a main problem. Spatial and social inequalities of health care remain. In the fifth section various aspects of drug use are examined. Health programmes are discussed such as the particular programme from mentally disadvantaged and the immunization programme.

Tackling health problems involves a human dimension. This means that besides the medical approach, also social, cultural, economic, and political factors have to be taken into account. For example, in health care planning, not only the physical accessibility is important, but economic, social, cultural and psychological factors influence the utilization of health services and medical consumption. The planning of health care delivery should take into account these elements. The contribution of medical geography has to be considered in the framework of health sciences in the perspective of applied medical geography. It can be a tool for health policy makers.

In disease ecology, the geographical approach consists of the spatial analysis of distribution patterns and the study of the relationship with environmental factors. Risk areas can be defined. Health, environment and development are intimately linked. The need for hygiene, sanitation and basic amenities is still a main concern in most of the developing countries. Health problems of the future should be faced. Growing life expectancy consequent upon the epidemiological transition will involve the problem of care for the elderly. The concept of avoidable deaths is worth considering. Disease control is not purely a matter of medical care. Multidisciplinary collaboration is necessary. We hope that this book will contribute to the goal of health for all.

Yola Verhasselt
Chair of the IGU Commission
on Health and Development

Acknowledgements

The editors are most grateful to individuals, agencies and organizations whose financial, material and moral support contributed to the huge success of the International Geographical Union (IGU) Commission on Health and Development Conference at the University of Ibadan in January 1992. We are indebted in particular to the Carnegie Corporation of New York, Commission of the European Community, the Nigerian Breweries Plc, Sterling Winthrop Plc, Lagos, the Commonwealth Foundation, the United States Agency for International Development (USAID) Lagos; the United Nations Population Fund (UNFPA), Lagos; Oyo State Government, Dunlop Nigeria Plc and Dr. Raymond Zard, Ibadan

We are also grateful to our contributors from around the world for making their research materials available and to our publisher, Avebury for positive consideration of the manuscript. Also we would like to thank Messrs E.E. Okoro, Braimah Saibu and Mrs. Yemisi Iwayemi for their editorial, indexing and endless typesetting.

1 Beyond health care delivery in Africa

Akin L. Mabogunje

Summary

The choice of topic is particularly appropriate at this time; for nothing shows more glaringly the weakness in the model of development that has been adopted in most African countries than the collapse in our ability to maintain ourselves in good health simply because of a drop, significant as this is, in the net export earnings of our various countries. In this presentation, therefore, I intend to argue that this collapse in the standard and quality of health of the masses of our population goes well beyond issues of financial resources and fiscal policies. It is, in fact, more the product of our inadequate appreciation of how most countries of Sub-Saharan African stand in the development process and what they should be doing to advance their present position and in the process improve the general health status of the majority of their population.

    The presentation is in five parts. The first part considers the current health situation in Africa and argues that the issue raised by this situation to be meaningful must be posited in the context of the political economy of the continent. The second part provides a brief digest of the political economy of Africa noting, in particular, the implication of the capitalist transformation initiated by colonialism for the aetiology and epidemiology of diseases on the continent. This leads to the third part which uses the concept of the social costs of production to show how the incompleteness of the colonially-induced capitalist transformation is at the root of the societal incapacity to improve on health conditions in Africa generally. The fourth part then proceeds to outline a strategy for advancing the process of capitalist transformation based on the strong community organisation on the continent but emphasizes the need to distinguish the concept of community from its somewhat casual use in health care delivery. A fifth and concluding section examines the range of health issues raised by this new perspective and shows how they in turn provide a fresh handle for deepening the development process at the grassroots level.

Akin L. Mabogunje

The health situation in Africa

Until recently, it was possible to conceptualize the health situation in most African countries largely in the context of an epidemiological transition model (Mosley et al, 1990). The model postulates a pre-transition phase in which the major health problems are those of infectious and parasitic diseases, nutritional deficiencies and reproductive health problems. These are gradually or dramatically resolved during a transition phase. They are then replaced in a post-transition phase by chronic and degenerative diseases of adult life such as cancer, stroke, lung and heart diseases, arthritis, and impairment of the nervous system.

In the context of this model, most sub-Saharan African countries have barely entered the transition phase. According to the World Bank report titled: *Sub-Saharan Africa: From Crisis to Sustainable Growth*, infectious and parasitic diseases dominate the health condition of a vast majority of the population. Infant mortality rates range between 100 and 170 for every 1,000 live births, compared with 33 and 32 in Sri Lanka and China respectively (The World Bank, 1989). In many of sub-Saharan African countries, deaths of children under five represent close to half of total deaths. In the poorest countries such as Niger, Mali, Burkina Faso and Ethiopia, only 70 to 77 per cent of children live to the age of five. Moreover, in 12 out of 29 countries for which data are available, the maternal mortality rate is higher than 500 for every 100,000 live births, compared with 44 in China and 90 in Sri Lanka. Each year, about 150,000 mothers in Africa die and roughly the same number suffer permanent disabilities because of complications from pregnancy and childbirth.

Since the late 1970s, with the economic crises and the structural adjustment programmes adopted to resolve these crises in most African countries, the health situation has worsened. Food availability has declined and the incidence of chronic malnutrition has risen sharply. This, along with the inadequate attention to reducing the high levels of fertility, has led to low birth-weight babies whose chances of withstanding infectious and parasitic diseases are consequently low. For those who survive these childhood diseases, morbidity rates remain high. It is estimated that some 200 million Africans (or nearly 45 per cent of the total) have chronic malaria and function under conditions of permanent health impairment. As a consequence, between 1979 and 1983 life expectancy declined in at least nine sub-Saharan African countries.

Even those countries where the health situation is not as grim, a growing burden of chronic and degenerative diseases, usually associated with health problems of industrialised countries is becoming increasing noticeable. On top of all this is the rapidly growing incidence of a devastating AIDS pandemic and other health threats such as those from drug addiction, environmental pollution and occupational hazards.

The health situation in most African countries is thus one of having, as it were, to cope simultaneously with two stages in the epidemiological transition model. Not unexpectedly, therefore, this double burden is straining the capabilities of the healthcare delivery

2

system in most of these countries almost to the point of collapse. It is this situation of acute break-down in the capacity of the health care delivery system that provokes an agonizing re-appraisal of the overall health situation and forces a return to fundamentals if we are eventually to find a way out of the labyrinth of conflicting strategies.

The most fundamental issue in this regard is, of course, to be clear what we mean by the word "health". According to the World Health Organisation, health is a state of complete physical, mental and social well-being and not merely the absence of disease and illness. This definition has been criticised as being an unwarranted abstraction since it alienates the health of an individual from the social context which determines it. This social context embraces not only socio-cultural practices and the environment but also the prevailing mode of production and State policy.

It is argued, for instance, that the incidence of schistosomiasis as a parasitic disease affecting individuals cannot be understood except in terms of a state policy that is remiss in providing adequate sanitation and water supplies for its citizens (Steven, 1985). Schistosomiasis is a disease for which snails are the intermediate hosts. It tends to spread easily and rapidly at large scale irrigation works where people live near snail-infested water. Proper measures can break the cycle of transmission and lower the incidence of infection. To do this, however, means that people living near irrigation ditches must be provided with adequate piped domestic water supply and enough latrines so as not to evacuate schistosome eggs into the water. The state engaging in construction of such major development works can factor these additional items into their costs. But the experience in most of Africa is that governments and aid donors usually underestimate the human costs of such projects and leave particularly the poorer classes in the region concerned to pay these costs in poor health and physical debilitation. A study in the late 1970s, of people living near the irrigation project in the Awash valley in Ethiopia, for instance, found that none of the farmers who benefitted from having irrigated plots in the settlement schemes within the project area was infected with the parasitic disease of schistosomiasis (Kloos, et al, 1981, 1979). However, 57 per cent of subsistence farmers crowded around the project, as well as an identical percentage of migrant labourers and their families who together constitute 90 per cent of the total population in the project area, were so infected.

In the same manner, the spread of malaria all across Africa in the 20th century can hardly be divorced from the colonial experience of African countries and the pattern of enclave development which it initiated. This pattern of development encouraged a widespread process of clearing forests and bush, and led to an increase in the percentage of *anopheles gambiae*, the most important malaria vector in the continent. In undisturbed forest, *anopheles gambiae* is one of the less common mosquito species. But, as different writers have noted, developmental activities of various types leading to forest clearing or accumulations of water tend to promote a very sharp rise in the number and areas occupied by the *anopheles gambiae*. In the Kano plains of Kenya, for instance, the initiation of the rice production scheme witnessed an increase in the population of *anopheles gambiae from one to 65 per cent of the total mosquito population (Hill et al, 1977).* Quarrying, mining, road construction and urban development all lead to earth movements and to small accumulations of water, with consequences of rapid expansion in the sway of the *anopheles gambiae* (Dutta *et al*. 1978).

According to Dunn, (1968) although the rates of prevalence and incidence of parasitic and infectious diseases are related to ecosystem diversity and complexity, the intensity of infection of sexually reproducing parasitic and infectious organisms rises sharply with ecosystem simplification and the creation of particularly uniform environment favourable for such organisms to achieve very high densities. This is because, although with such simplification, there are fewer species of potential intermediate hosts for parasitic and infectious organisms, the process of indirect disease transmission tends to become more highly efficient. It is such ecosystem simplification, resulting from the creation of man-made lakes which provide the environments of worms and snails to reproduce easily and to intensify the incidence of schistosomiasis. Similarly, forest clearing and large-scale commercial agriculture create suitable environments for the anopheles gambiae and thus promotes the areal scope and intensity of malarial infection.

It is of course, unconscionable to argue from this that developmental activities are antithetical to the maintenance of a healthy environment. What these illustrations do, is to put in sharper focus the dominant role of political economy embracing both State policy and the prevailing mode of production in any consideration of health issues. For it is political economy that explains, for instance, why in Africa, none of the authorities - colonial, national and international - have been able to engage in a full-scale campaign at malaria eradication. As Hedman and others indicated, even in a holo-endemic region such as Liberia, significant achievement in malaria eradication was possible when the mining company operating in the area was determined to commit adequate resources to this goal (Hedman *et al;* 1979). Although the estimated cost of the control programme (which was put at US$4.00 per person) was considered an underestimate, the crucial fact is that when authorities decide to pay the costs, real gains can be made in promoting healthy situations. In order therefore to appreciate the close relation between health issues and political economy, it is necessary to explore briefly the significant elements in the colonial transformation of African economy and society in the first six decades of this century.

Health and Africa's political economy

The advent of colonialism in Africa represents a major watershed not only in the socio-economic situation of the continent but also in the aetiology and epidemiology of diseases. Before the colonial era, the prevailing mode of production over large parts of the continent can best be described as pre-capitalist. Within this system of production, kinship relations were the dominant factor for articulating and co-ordinating all societal activities. Kinship determines the individual's access to the various factors of production, notably labour, land, credit and enterprise. For example, in a pre-capitalist and pre-colonial

Nigeria, where you lived, whether in a town or in the rural area, what work you do, your claim to any plot of land for farming or building and even the skills you are allowed to acquire - all these are a function of whose son or daughter you are. It is thus easy to appreciate that your health status would, to a large extent, be dependent on your kinship relationship so far as this determines your nutritional status through the size of family labour and family land to which individual has access.

But, more importantly, the dominance of kinship relations in the political economy means that territoriality rather than mobility was the paramount feature of social life. Most people do not move far from their home base. Except for long-distance traders, the warriors and the slaves, the majority of the population live out their lives within an environment they had learnt to relate to and to depend upon for their health needs. Whenever there was some upsurge in the incidence of particular disease or when, through climatic variability, there was famine and widespread hunger, the societies had institutional mechanisms for sharing and thus for reducing the burden of these events on the health of individuals. This is not to say that inadequate knowledge of disease vectors, defective nutritional balance and variable attention to environmental sanitation did not give rise to significant rates of morbidity and mortality at the level of individual households. But if the truth be told, we probably know less about health conditions in those distant pasts than our speculative scholarship would admit. Or, as Feierman (1985) would put it: "Quite probably the seasonal malnutrition which is so important a part of the health picture in today's Africa did not exist then. It is remarkable that after decades of mature scholarship on African history we are ignorant on so fundamental an issue" (Steven Feierman, 1985).

At any rate, one of the most important missions of colonialism was to terminate this mode of production and to replace kinship relations with the money nexus as the coordinating factor in social relations. Indeed, the colonial mission in Africa was to penetrate the pre-capitalist economies dominant over large areas of the continent and to transform and integrate them into the global free market capitalist economy. Although the word "capitalism" has come to acquire strong negative connotations in most colonial territories, it is important to stress that little attention has been paid to understanding its real essence in most of these countries. For, whatever may be said about capitalism, it has proved in human history to be far the most effective mode of production for generating and accumulating tremendous material wealth in any given society.

To do this, however, capitalism requires that a society must arrange its affairs such that every societal resource, whether of labour, land, capital or entrepreneurship, must be brought to the free market and given a price tag as if it were a mere commodity (Polauyi, 1957). Commoditizing societal resources is, however, a process of singular difficulty, but this is at the very core of economic growth and development. For instance, to commoditize land involves tremendous activities of individualising the ownership of land, surveying its unit parts, and setting up systems of adjudication, registration and titling. For the developed countries, these critical sets of activities that were required to propel their societies into the free market economy took decades of determined effort to accomplish. Similarly, commoditizing human labour meant compelling individuals through taxation and various devices including hunger and destitution to go out and sell their labour for a wage. It is so easy to forget that in traditional societies every individual was self-employed. No one puts himself out as seeking wage employment. Receiving wages for labour is part of the capitalist transformation of pre-capitalist societies. With it also came the notion of unemployment and poverty. Capital, either in the form of credit, professional knowledge, technical know-how or machinery and equipment also became commoditized with a price tag in the form of interest rates or user fees. The enterprising effort of entrepreneurs, in turn is priced as a commodity in the size of profit that accrues to his effort.

The consequences of the colonial effort to transform African economies and societies from the pre-capitalist to the capitalist were evident in the changed geography of the continent. The enclave plantation, export agriculture, mining and transportation activities changed the environmental conditions over sizeable areas. The need of these activities for wage labour called into existence large streams of labour migrants moving from one part of the continent to another. The agglomeration of significant number of these migrants at particular locations led to the growth of urban centres. The failure of an increasing number of such migrants to secure gainful employment in the cities initiated an era of shanty housing with few infrastructural facilities and poor environmental sanitation. Their migration away from the rural areas, in turn, meant the loss of a significant section of the economically active population with negative consequences for family life, social collective effectiveness, economic vitality and adequate environmental control.

These tendencies initiated in the colonial period have by and large been continued and actively promoted in all the post-colonial states in Africa. For a significant proportion of the African population, this exposure of socio-economic life to the operations of the free-market forces with its emphasis on the money nexus has meant serious dislocation and the undermining of the integrity of the social life to which they were accustomed. The extensive mobility which had become the order of the day greatly changed the epidemiology of diseases over large areas of the continent. Professor Mansell Prohero study of Migrants and Malaria remains a classic in its clarity and insightfulness.

However, as Polanyi rightly observed, one of the characteristics of capitalism is that where free market forces are allowed to operate unrestrained, they have a tendency to dislocate and undermine the integrity of social life. As such as a society becomes capitalistic, it tends to erect certain institutional protections such as trade unionism, factory regulations, legal contract and other statutory limitations on the operations of the market to ensure the well-being and welfare of the citizen. Such protections do entail costs and can thus be regarded as the social costs of capitalist production. This concept of the social costs of any mode of production is of vital significance for appreciating the health status of any society at any given point of time. For this reason, it will be necessary to elaborate a little further on the concept.

Health and the social costs of production

According to Feierman (1985), the social costs of production refer to the costs of making working conditions healthy. It includes the costs of feeding workers and their families, of maintaining retired workers, and of either controlling or containing the environmental effects of the production process. In the context of a capitalist mode of production, question as to who should pay these costs or how these should be distributed are relevant not only for understanding the fate of those employed for wages but also for peasant producers who may benefit from extension services, public education and health services. They are also vital for appreciating the circumstances of those who may be compelled to produce cash crops at price levels which only hasten the descent to poverty and misery, and for people who happen by chance to live near fields sprayed by harmful pesticides. In other words, trying to understand the social costs of production makes it possible to identify political and economic decisions which have an impact on the distribution of sickness and death - decisions, for example, on whether to invest in sanitation, education, health care and family support.

The concept of the social costs of production thus enables us to better appreciate the relation between health issues, the prevailing mode of production and the adequacy of State policy in erecting necessary institutional protection against the consequences of the unrestrained operations of free market forces. Reference has already been made to how far the widespread incidence of schistosomiasis and malaria infection can be largely attributed to the inadequacy of State policy. This inadequacy can also be shown to have been critical for the health of women and children. It has been remarked, for instance, that the colonial and post-colonial bias towards export and commercial agricultural production, which is usually undertaken by men, had resulted in credit and extension services being directed only towards them whilst women's farming for food crops is treated as uneconomic subsistence activity. Yet, there are indications that over the past century the displacement of male labour from food production has drastically affected the organization of women's work and the distribution of their work time, with significant consequences for maternal and child malnutrition.

With much of the responsibility for subsistence farming falling on women, their nutrition and that of their children suffers tremendously, especially during the season of peak demand for agricultural labour. Schofield for instance, in his survey of the effects of seasonal labour peaks on child nutrition noted that at this season women prepare meals less frequently; have less time to gather green leafy vegetables, often leave the cooking pot to simmer for too long thus destroying vitamins, come home to cook after the children have fallen asleep, generally do less house keeping, limit fuel and water collection and, on the whole, devote less time to their children's care (Hull, *et al*; 1933). The women themselves often go hungry during this period, which is towards the end of the rainy season when the previous year's food is nearly exhausted and the new year's crops have not yet matured.

Nutritional levels during this hungry season seriously determine the disease picture in most of rural Africa. It is reported, for instance, that 78 per cent of childhood deaths in the Gambia in 1964 occurred during the rainy season (Onchere *et al.* 1964). Diarrhoea, which is one of the commonest causes of children morbidity and mortality in Africa, tends to affect more children during this hungry rainy season. Yet, there are indications that the situation had not always been like this. The increasing monetization of the economy has meant that the old system of hungry season sharing has declined and is being replaced by a new system in which the poor borrow money during the hungry season to buy food, become indebted to those better off, have even greater difficulty meeting the exigencies of the next hungry season and eventually lose their land and their self-employment capability.

Within a fullblown capitalist system, payment for these social costs of production are widely distributed and are usually borne by the State, by corporate capital, by the consumers and to some extent by the workers themselves through contributions to social security schemes. Sometimes these social costs are paid through health insurance schemes subsidized by employers or by the State or by the afflicted and often cover all members of the family including women and children. Thus, although a system of individualised health care provided by priced professionalized services is the order in these societies, its efficiency and effectiveness can be appreciated only in the context of the social relations of capitalist production in which everything has been commoditized and monetized.

The problem in most African countries, however, is that, in spite of nearly a century of colonial and post-colonial efforts of governments, the transition from pre-capitalist to a capitalist mode of production has been blocked. The colonial state and, to date its *independent* national successor, failed totally to extinguish and replace the social relations of pre-capitalist societies in most parts of Africa. Everywhere, the peasants and their pre-capitalist mode of production remain in some form of accommodation within a free market economy. Workers have not been totally converted into a proletariat with their labour as the only resource available to them to sell. Land has not been totally individualised and commoditized. Kinship relations still dominate large areas of social life and the money nexus has failed to determine access to all of societal resources. In short, as Lonsdale observed, "capitalism was weak in Africa", its productive efficiency contested by pre-capitalist forms whose reproductive costs were not a liability in the market. The power of colonial states did bring capitalism closer to the point of production ... (but) colonialism could not cope with a capitalist transaction (Lonsdale, 1981).

The result is a political economy described as one of "syncretic articulation", an economy of uneven and combined development with both capitalist and pre-capitalist features. This type of economy is this one where the locus of computation of the social costs of production remains indeterminate as between kinship institutions and market-related State programmes. This indeterminacy is thus the central problem of health administration and health care delivery in most of Africa. Put in this way, it is thus easy to see why the resolution of the health crisis in most African countries can only happen in the context of a strategy of development that moves African countries towards completing their transition to full-blown free market economies. The possibility of such a strategy of development is entailed in a focus on the community as an institution. It is argued that the transformation or radicalization of this institution holds the key not only for more rapid development but also for vastly improved health status for the majority of the African population.

Health, development and the community

The idea that much in the present situation of health care delivery can be improved if the community can be made to participate more actively in the process is becoming part of a new orthodoxy in the health profession. This is seen as particularly important if primary health care were to be extended to a large section of the population and their access to basic health services enhanced. The position was succinctly put by the World Bank as follows:

> Safeguarding budget allocations for health care, especially for the provision of primary health care, is essential if health services are to achieve their potential contributions to improved health, productivity and development. These might be best accomplished in many African countries if people, individuals, families and communities - take the responsibility for their own health care. Government, NGOs and the private sector need to provide support for these efforts. Communities must be consulted and encouraged to participate in setting their own priorities and in the design and delivery of health programmes (The World Bank, 1989).

The critical issue here, however, is that community is often used as a rather casual and at best topographic concept to refer to a group of people, may be occupying a definable territory. Such a concept is perhaps valid in the context of healthcare delivery when the emphasis is on some episodic ministration such as innoculation or vaccination. It is less meaningful or valid in the context of development or sustainable health care programming. For the concept to have a high degree of realism, it is vital to position it in the context of social relations that is in the process of being transformed with changes in the prevailing mode of production. In other words, in most of Africa, we are confronted with community organisations within which, although kinship ties remain relatively strong, they are in various stages of being replaced by social relations based increasingly on the money nexus. This nexus, however, has three dimensions of relevance within a community. These are the productive, the social class and the political dimension.

The productive dimension relates to the degree to which the allocative processes of productive resources in a society are governed by exchange rather than use consideration. In the African context, the dimension entails, for instance, that market forces have overturned traditional African tenure system and subverted the traditional family control on labour. The social class dimension, on the other hand, emphasizes the extent to which society has become polarised as between those who own capital and those who have to sell their labour for wages. The political dimension indicates the extent to which the conflictual tension inherent in the relation between these two classes in society fosters and sustains democratic tendencies by forcing a break with ascriptive determinants of access to power and influence within the given society.

These three dimensions of the social relations embedded in the money nexus help to underscore the ambivalence still characteristic of social relations in community organisations in most of Africa due to the incomplete nature of the transition to a free market economy (Lonsdale, 1981). To a large extent, this incompleteness of transition is responsible for the difficulty of sustaining many health care efforts based on community organisations in the continent. The difficulties of mobilizing communities for self-help around health-related projects such as water and sanitation schemes are daunting enough but they can be and often have been surmounted. In many African countries such a mobilised effort has been induced and initiated by various external donor agencies and non-governmental organisations. However, it is generally acknowledged that to sustain interest in and, in particular, to manage and maintain such projects in good repair over time requires the routine mobilization and availability of community resources on a continuing basis. The experience of community management of rural water supply and sanitation services in six countries, four of which are in Africa (Sierra Leone, Togo, Malawi and Kenya) underscores this point. The most successful and most sustainable of these schemes was that of the Kwale district in Kenya where "the communities themselves manage and finance the pumps. (Moreover), because of the close tie between health education and community development, links have been established that make it easier to co-ordinate and organize multi-sectoral teams of extension agents" (McCommon *et al;* 1990).

The realization of the layered and multi-dimensional nature of the concept of community organisation focuses attention back to the role of the State in the development process. It emphasizes that the community as a social institution, properly identified, mobilized and "radicalized" represents the veritable unit that must be transformed if the whole nation is to be developed. Seeing the community as an institution allows us better to appreciate how it can be transformed or "radicalized". Institutions have been defined as "a set of rules, the enforcement characteristics of those rules and the norms of behaviour that are sustained by those rules in repeated human interactions" (North 1989). These three elements that define any institution, that is, rules, enforcement characteristics and norms of behaviour, have been noticed not to change at the same pace. The rules are more likely to be changed rapidly by various decisions or practices but the enforcement characteristics and the norms of behaviour change at relatively slower pace. It is this variation in the pace of change of institutional elements that explains why there is the appearance of so much continuity even in a period of most revolutionary changes. Thus, "radicalization" of an institution such as a community means changing some of its rules of operation whilst still capitalizing on its enforcement capabilities and the norms of behaviour these sustain (Mabogunje, 1991).

The mobilization and radicalization of the community as an institution has been the principle underlying a new strategy of development. Although such institutional radicalization has been going on for a long time and has been used for real developmental effect (notice the important role of Town Unions or Community Development Associations in the provision of vital infrastructural facilities in their communities), it is only recently that the process is being elevated to the status of a national strategy of development. In Nigeria, the last six years have witnessed a quite impressive developmental impact arising from the adoption of this strategy. The setting up of a Directorate of Food, Roads and Rural Infrastructures, of the Better Life Programme for Rural Women and the more recent inauguration of Community Banks all have as their basic objective the mobilization and radicalization of the community through changing the rules concerning forms of productive organizations within the community, modes of ensuring and enhancing access of small producers to credit, the rate at which the economy at the level of community is being monetized and the range and types of infrastructural facilities available for the community over large areas of the country. All of these are meant to weaken significantly the sway of the pre-capitalist relations of production and to pave the way for the full flowering of the free market forces in generally determining social relations at this very grass-root level.

The structural adjustment programme that most African economies have been subjected to over the last decade can thus be seen as the consequences of the contradictions inherent in the syncretic nature of the economy which we inherited from colonial times and which we have not been sufficiently perceptive or successful in fully transforming. That transformation or the "unblocking" of the process of transition to the free market economy has now been forced on us almost willy-nilly. It is, however, not too clear that we are getting correctly the message of the times or that, when we are, we are seizing the tacticals advantages presented by the current situation. This would appear particularly so in respect of the health conditions of the majority of the people in most African countries. In the concluding part of this paper, therefore, I wish to raise what I consider the critical issues of health care delivery posed by the current status of the development process in most African countries.

Conclusion

Clearly, to pose the question: "what are the health issues in development?" is to primarily ask how can African peoples keep themselves in relatively good health whilst their society is undergoing the strains and stresses of development. Framed in this way, this question makes the issue of how much is spent on the purchase of drugs, how many hospitals are available in the country, how many doctors or nurses are there per 100,000 of the population and similar ratios and indicators, although important, of a second order of relevance. The question as framed thus ensures that we see health rather than its negation, for what it is, that is, the autonomous ability of individuals to cope with their environment on a continuing basis.

Against, this background therefore, I would want to put forward the following seven issues as worthy of concern in the circumstances.

First, what societal organisational arrangements do we put in place to ensure that the environment is less disease-ridden and more conducive to promoting healthy living on a continuous and sustainable basis in different African countries? The thrust of this paper is to challenge the casual use of the concept of community. The issue remains how well has the traditional community as a unit of societal organisation survived in different African countries? Can it be mobilised and radicalized to serve the complementary purpose of development and good health?

Secondly, within such a community organisation, how do we enhance the access of the individual to the information and enlightenment resources needed to raise his consciousness and his capacity to maintain a healthy life-style and sustain his good health? The issue here is not only of health education but involves health counselling and a formalised social programmes of health activities of the type so familiar with the Chinese. Whilst this does not exclude curative health-care, it puts in the context of a safety-net needed when there are unavoidable breakdowns in the health of individuals.

Thirdly, how do we ensure that the individual, particularly when a mother or a child, has access to the variety and quantity of food items that can ensure adequate and qualitatively appropriate nutrition on a continuing and sustainable basis? Subsistence agriculture belongs in part to the persistence of a pre-capitalist economy in most African countries. But, as Feierman observed, there are compelling evidence suggesting that under the impact of the syncretic articulation of today's economy fewer varieties of food crops are being cultivated by rural households practising subsistence agriculture today than say a hundred years ago. Yet, the market in food commodities is as yet so inadequately developed in many countries to make up for this loss of variety and balance. Indeed, the study of food markets in most African countries is seldom treated as an aspect of health and yet it is central to the whole issue of malnutrition and poor health for a large proportion of the population.

Fourthly, how do we ensure that within the family context, the number of children is kept within the limit that can be effectively nurtured and catered for whilst the mother's health is also appropriately sustained? The issue here is the problem of striking on a chord that can give the appropriate social resonance on this issue. The situation in most African countries is one of conflicting signals. Religion, tradition and the strong survival of the kinship safety net make family planning not such a compelling necessity. What type of countervailing factors other than publicity and policy pronouncements give greater force, at least to the health advantages of small families?

Fifthly, how do we reduce, contain or obviate man-made hazards that are the concomitants of the very process of development? Some of the issues of soil erosion land degradation, deforestation, ecosystem simplification and so on are well-known as well as their consequences for nutritional levels and susceptibility to disease vectors of various kinds. More recently, there is, in addition, an increasing range of technological hazards and toxic pollutions to which African countries are being unwittingly exposed. Again, the issue here is one not only of awareness but also of an organised capacity at the level of communities or groups of communities to protect or resist such unwarranted assault on their health conditions. How can such a capacity be built up given the limited level of formal education in the society.

Sixthly, when health actually breaks down, how do we ensure that the drugs and medications required to restore health are easily accessible to all? The issue here is not just one of meeting the high cost of importation or of dispensing drugs. It relates to how the herbal and other curative resources available within a given country can be relatively cheaply garnered, processed and utilised in appropriate doses for the health care of the majority. This issue calls attention also to the need for a more creative and realistic strategy of collecting, systematising, validating and popularising traditional knowledge and systems of coping with certain diseases and ailments for which so-called traditional healers or "witch-doctors" are the repository in most African countries.

Seventhly, how does the State provide the enabling and supportive environment which would encourage the communities to take major responsibility for the provision, management and maintenance of infrastructural facilities and health-care delivery systems that it needs to ensure a high health status for all of its members? The issue here also relates to those of administrative decentralisation and democratic governance at the grassroots. The experience in most African countries is that administrative decentralisation has many and different meaning to those in power and authority. But, more importantly, democratic governance, whilst it may be sweeping across the continent at the level of central governments, is still a highly contested issue at the grassroots levels. Even if there is no contest and democratic governance is permitted to operate at the level of the grassroots, it is important to remember that, given the strongly syncretic nature of social relations at his level, and the persistent importance of the ascriptive factor in these relations, there is need for a serious effort at capacity building at the level of the ordinary citizens to ensure that they understand and will defend the need for transparency, accountability and sustainability in running community services either for health purposes or for development.

These seven issues shown in each case how difficult it is to attempt to isolate problems of healthcare delivery from the socio-economic context in which they are deeply embedded. This, of course, is not to say that health issues cannot be tackled on their own merit. Indeed, this has been the pattern of healthcare delivery services in most African countries to date. What, however, can be said is that for the issues that they raise to be tackled in an effective manner or for health care delivery systems to be sustainable in the long-term requires that health care be conceived of as part of the development process in a country. This means that healthcare delivery agencies would do well to appreciate the tactical advantages of focusing on the community as the unit of operational mobilisation. It also entails that they recognise that if these tactical advantages were not used to promote a more far-reaching strategy of developmental transformation in the community the efficiency of the health care delivery system itself may stall and falter. It is thus the hope that the present text will help to clarify and articulate the many different ways in which health care activities and developmental processes can be made mutually reinforcing and tremendously productive of material wealth and a higher quality of life for the majority of the population in most African countries and indeed most third world countries.

References

Dunn, F.L. (1968). 'Epidemiological factors health and disease in hunter gatherers', in Lee, R.B. and de vore, I. (eds), man the hunter, Chicago: Aldine.

Dutta, H.M. and Dutt, A.K. (1978). 'Malaria Ecology: A Global Perspective'. *Social Science and Medicine*, 12: 69-84

Feiermam S. (1985). Struggles for Control: The social roots of health and healing in modern Africa. *African Studies Review* 28, 2/3: 96.

Headman, P., Brohult, J., Forlund, J., Sirleaf, Vaud Bengtssom, E. (1979). 'A pocket of controlled malaria in a holoendemic region of West Africa; Annals of Tropical Medicine and Parasitology, 73/4. :317-325.

Hill, M.N., Chandler, J.A. and Highton, R.R. (1977). 'A comparison of mosquito population in irrigated and non-irrigated areas of the Kano plains, Nyanza Province, Kenya, in Worthington, E.B. (ed) Arid Land Irrigation in Developing Countries: Environmental Problems and Effects, Oxford: Pergamon Press.

Hull, H.F., Williams, P.J. and Oldfield, F. 'Measles mortality and vaccine efficiency in rural West Africa" *Lancet* 972-75

Kloos, H., Desole, G. and Lemma, A. (1981). Intestinal parasitism in seminomadic pastoralists and subsistence farmers in and around irrigation schemes in the Awash Valley, Ethiopia, with special emphasis on ecological and cultural associations'. *Social Science and Medicine*, 15B: 457-69.

Kloos, H. and Thompson, K .(1979). 'Schistosomiasis in Africa: an ecological perspective'. *Journal of Tropical Geography, 48, 31-46.*

Londale, J. (1981). 'States and social processes in Africa: historiographical survey' African Review 24, 2/3: 190-191.

Mabogunje, A. (1991). 'A new paradigm for urban development strategy in developing countries'. World Bank Annual Conference in Development Economics, Washington D.C.

McCommon, C., Warner, D. and Yohalem, D. (1990). 'Community management of rural water supply and sanitation services, UNDP, World Bank Water and Sanitation Programme, WASH Technical Report, 67: Washington 22-23.

Mosley, W.H., Jamison, D.T. and Henderson, D.A. (1990). 'The health sector in developing countries: problems for the 1990s and beyond'. *Annual Review of Public Health*, 11:

North, D.C. (1989). 'Institutions and economic growth: a historical introduction', World Development, 17; (19) 1319-1332.

Onchere, S.R. and Sloof, R. (1981). 'Nutrition and diseases in machakos district Kenya', in Chambers, R., Longhurst, R. and Pacey, A. (eds.) Seasonal Dimensions of Rural Poverty, London: Frances Pinter.

Polauyi, K. (1957). 'The Great transformation.' The political and economic origins of our time, Boston: Beacon Press.

Schofield, S. (1974). 'Seasonal factors', Journal of Development Studies, 11:(1) 22-40.

World Bank (1989). Sub-Saharan African: From Crisis to Sustainable Growth: A long Term Perspective Study, Washington D.C.

Part I
HEALTH CONSEQUENCES OF ENVIRONMENTAL CHANGES

Introduction

Susana I. Curto de Casas

We can consider that disease is man's answer to environmental stimuli only. However it is the most important answer, because human existence and the species survival depends on it.

Health and diseases have accompanied men through history. The history of human health, diseases and death is dynamic, evolving with economic and social changes because the environment does not solely consist of physical and biological factors, it includes cultural, economic and social conditions. For example, prehistoric remains of people who lived in Glacial Ages present signs of chronic osteoarthrosis, may be as a consequence of living in wet and dark caverns. But centuries after, in the Middle Ages, plague and its agents invaded Europe introduced by commercial trade with the Orient opened by the Crusades. As a consequence of these epidemics a large period of demographic decrease began, agricultural decline and economic recession forced people to eat the contaminated which was lying on the ground and so started epidemics of ergotism.

In the 19th century, tuberculosis has been linked to unhealthy urban conditions during the Industrial Revolution. Today respiratory diseases are growing due to polluted air. A modern life style produces stress and increases the incidence of cardiovascular diseases. Tobacco, alcohol, drugs promiscuity are health problems in modern societies.

Environmental changes transform the disease ecology, in consequence the knowledge of environmental factors and physiological responses of humans is essential to humanity, and the answers to these questions have been searched for by man since remote times.

In the past, environmental changes occurred at local scale, but nowadays they have regional and global dimensions such as Amazonian deforestation, ocean pollution, atmospheric heating, urbanization, agricultural changes or modern communication systems. In consequence, diseases can be diffused by countries and continents, through different social classes, income levels and developed status.

This part includes papers with different geographical approaches to the influence of environmental changes on health, at various scales.

Changes in global climate will represent a rapid change in the global environment. Its effects on human health will be most important in some areas of the Third World because it could have influence on the ecology of some insects, vectors of endemic diseases and could affect the diseases diffusion and control plans. Curto de Casas et al; analyze the future geographical distribution of malaria and Chagas disease in Argentina using analogic and stimulation models of probable regional climate changes produced by the global warming.

Man-made changes in landscapes produce a variety of impacts on the endemic diseases foci functioning. The assessment of the impact of agriculture on natural endemic diseases in Africa is a problem of medical geography approached by S. Malkhazova and T. Yu. Karimova using statistical analysis and forecasting. Agricultural production with more intensive development of farming may entail substantial changes in the environment and so, the foci of diseases that exist in natural landscapes could be transformed as a result of changes in ecosystems due to agricultural land use or by changes in the contacts with the population involved. The small-scale study of the area could provide additional information about the nature of the difficult issue concerning disease predictions.

Changes in economic development are related with the diminishing of two Chinese endemic diseases. Tan Jian an et al relate the decline of the incidence of Keshan disease and Kaschin-Beck disease in regions with low selenium in the ecosystem, to the improvement of selenium by the trade of new crops and a change in the population diet.

Changes in economic and social activities could influence health communities by producing a variation in the incidence of some endemic diseases. Gustave Yameogo's paper analyses the variation of prevalence of dracunculosis in function of different months of the year and correlated it with the intensity of agricultural works and population age in the South West of Burkina Faso.

Health is recognized as a crucial component of development, but development often results in unexpected changes in the environment, and the environment, in return, may create new health hazards. Geographers have a duty to anticipate the likely outputs in order to improve plans and policies in health prevention. This part is a good example of the geographical contribution to these health studies.

2 Global distribution of American pathogenic complexes

Susana I. Curto de Casas, Juan J. Burgos, Rodolfo U. Carcavallo, Carlos Mena Segura and Maria de Los Angeles Y. Lopez

Summary

This paper updates the knowledge about the present geographical distribution of two vectors of important South American endemies and the bioclimatic factors which are associated with them.

One of the species is *A. darlingi*, a predominantly wild vector of malaria and the other is *T. infestans* a predominantly domestic vector of American Trypanosomiasis (Chagas disease). In both cases, the studies applied analogical and stimulation models of the most relevant probable climatic changes to identify the factors influencing their diffusion.

The results of our analysis indicate that climatic factors influence the spatial diffusion of *A. darlingi*, while *T. infestans* is strongly influenced by the overpopulation density growth.

Introduction

The geographic distribution of the vectors of important South American diseases is related to bioclimatic factors; some of them, like temperature and rainfall, can be measured with statistical association.

The global climate change predicted for the near future will produce a greenhouse influence which may increase the temperature and thereby change the amount and distribution of rainfall. These effects will be important in the geographical distribution of vegetation and animal, including vectors and hosts of human diseases.

This paper analyzes the geographical distribution of *Anopheles (N) darlingi* and *Triatoma infestans*, malaria and Chagas disease vectors in Argentina, some predicted climate changes and their influence on the vectors.

Material and method

The analysis of the geographical distribution of vectors is based on literature review and fieldwork. The latter was made for the North West only, so this paper uses information from the scientific literature.

The information of *A. (N) darlingi* is from Bejarano (1959 and 1971) Mitchel and Darsie (1985) and the National Service of malaria Control (Senapa, 1991).

The information on *T. infestans* is from Bejarano (1967), Carcavallo and Martinez (1968), Martinez and Chichero (1972), Carcavallo (1976), Curto de Casas (1983 and 1991), Curto de Casas and Carcavallo (1984), Canale and Carcavallo (1985, Carcavallo, Becker, Canale and Rozemwurcel (1988).

The global climate changes uses the NCAR predictions: Community Climate Models, from the National Centre of Atmospheric Research, Boulder, Colorado, USA, (Washington and Meehl, 1983 and 1984), 9 atmospheric layers, and GISS model predictions: Goddar Institute of Space and Science, New York, USA, (Hansen et al, 1984 and 1987), 9 atmospheric layers, and the variations proposed by Burgos, Fuenzalida Ponce and Molion (1991) introduced by Amazonia Basin deforestation.

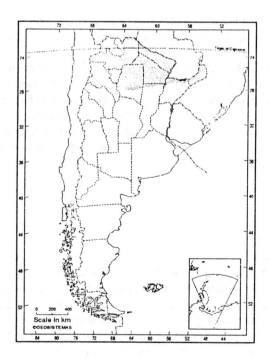

Figure 2.1   **Anopheles (N) darlingi [Geographical Distribution]**

Geographical distribution of vectors

A. darlingi has been found in the northern provinces of Salta Jujuy, Formosa, Chaco, Santiago de Estero, Misiónes and Corrientes (Fig 2.1).

According to Bejarano (1971) its presence in Argentina is irregular, with great variations in time and space. Only in few instances was it found in consecutive years in the same place. Exceptionally, it arrived in the NW and the dry lands of Chaco. The Guayra Fall (Brazil) is the southern limit of the permanent presence of this species.

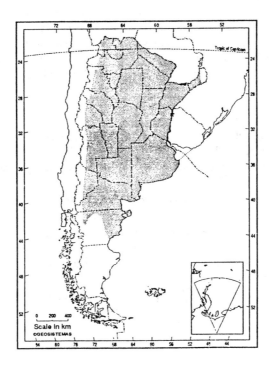

Figure 2.2   Triatoma infestans [geographical distribution]

T. infestans is found in all regions of Argentina, from the north to Caleta Cordova (46°S) and from the sea to the high altitude of the Andes (highest alt. is Cienaguillas, 3642 m) with the exception of the NE of Misiones and Somuncura plateau in Chubut (Fig. 2.2).

23

Bioclimatic factors

A. darlingi.

It lives in the subtropical rainfall forest, dry tropical forest and subtropical savannas. The felling of trees in the Chaco dry forest diminishes the local evapotranspiration and saturates the subterranean water. In consequence, rain water pools stay for long periods.

According to Bejarano (1971) it is a wild and anthropozootic species, which develops its larvae in partially shady, static or flowing waters, with water vegetation. In Misiones they grow in small streams flowing into the Parana river and flooded waterside places.

Until 1965, its presence on the Parana shores in Misiones coincided with rainy periods, which produced floods in terrain without slopes. Since 1965, the endemicity disappeared from Misiones until 1989, when it arrived having been preceded by great number of cases in the border area of Paraguay and Brazil, but it was not found on the Argentinean shore of the Parana river (Senapa, 1991). Its presence in Paraguay and Brazillian shore of Parana river was imputed due to 38 new great dams built in the Southern Parana basin, which reproduces the ecological environment of the species (Curto de Casas and Boffi, 1990).

T. infestans:

It had high infestation in the dry tropical forest (Chaco), xerophytic forest, thornbush forest, NW foothills and valleys, NW desert plateau, and less infestation in the eastern subtropical forest, western subtropical forest, central savanna (pampas) and Patagonian plains.

According to Bejarano (1971) it is adapted to all climates. Notwithstanding this, it prefers dry climates, but it develops well in laboratories at 70% humidity. When the environment is drier, it eats more and in consequence the population density grows.

Hack (1955) noted a shorter cycle with higher temperatures. In consequence, he inferred that in hot regions there would be two generations per year.

Jorg (1962) observed that it does not eat when the temperature is below $10^{o}C$, and Hack (1955) noted that it did not moult when the temperature is below 7 to $9^{o}C$.

Blaksley and Carcavallo (1968) conducted experiments which verified that 88% of adults survived 4 hours at $-2^{o}C$. and 50% survived more than 1 hour at $-6^{o}C$.

According to Aragao (1971) it lives in moderate temperatures. The observation is confirmed by the triatomine disappearance in the Central Patagonian Plateau, which has lower temperatures.

Curto de Casas (1983) associated the geographical distribution of T. infestans and its infestation degree, with the number of days with more than $20^{o}C$, and the annual amount of air saturation deficit. So, the southern limit of the species is not given by minimum temperatures, but for the few days with higher temperatures (Curto de Casas and Carcavallo, 1984).

High temperatures would accelerate the metabolism, and air saturation deficit would increase the necessity of food by thirst. Both conditions, would produce an accelerated moulting and high population densities as a consequence.

Global climate change

Two decades ago, some models had evaluated the global increase of temperature produced by increase of atmospheric CO_2 and other greenhouse gases. The predictions change according to the model numerical models based on a tridimensional analysis of the atmospheric thermodynamics and the ocean surface in contact, predict an increase of global temperature and rainfall, but they show discrepancies at a regional or local scale.

The NCAR and GISS are the models which predict the greatest climate changes with less errors in the world over the last 100 years.

If these predictions would have occurred, the increase of mean temperature in the central part of South America would have exceeded $+1^{o}C$ in 2010 and $+2.5^{o}C$ in 2050 in the Pampas region and savannas trough of central western Argentina.

Fig. 2.4 shows the rainfall GISS and NCAR predictions for December-January-February and June-July-August.

Predictions for Argentinean climates are a subtropical climate in the Pampa ($+1$ or $+2.5^{o}C$ temperature increase and 10% more rainfall) and drier in the central and western regions (high temperature, with similar or less amount of rainfall). (Fig. 2.5)

The vegetative covering dynamics is an important change factor in South America, but it has not been considered in the GCCh models. Molion (1988) has established a preliminary prediction of climate change, describing the change in the subcontinent with an increase of CO_2 with and without deforestation. The pattern of the change is shown in Fig. 2.6.

Fig. 2.6 shows in (A) the possible changes without deforestation: a north-south wetter-drier-wetter configuration, and in (B) the possible changes with a large scale deforestation scenario of a north-south drier-wetter-drier configuration.

Discussion and conclusion

In the hypothesis of a stable climate, the geographical distribution of vector species can be changed in two ways: (a) diminishing the area and population densities, and (b) increasing them.

(a)   produced by different man-made controls to improve the environment and to reduce the epidemiological risk conditions like insecticides, biological-genetic techniques, sanitary engineering, for example the programmes of malaria or yellow fever control at a national level in some countries.

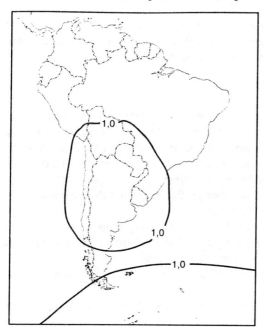

2010 s

Increase in $^{\circ}$C in the decadal mean temperature (Hansen et al, 1987 and 1988).

2050 s

Increase in oC in the decadal mean temperature (Hansen et al, 1987 and 1988).

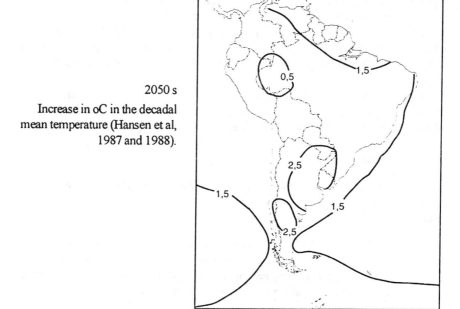

Figure 2.3   Temperature of surface (GISS MODEL)

Dec-Jan-Feb   June-Jul-Aug

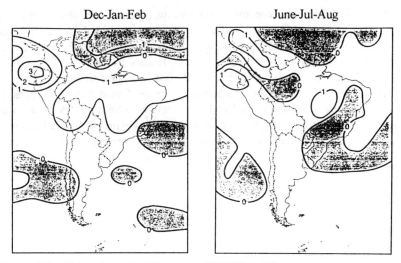

Figure 2.4a   Values for rainfall changes [GISS Model]

Dec-Jan-Feb   Jun-Jul-Aug

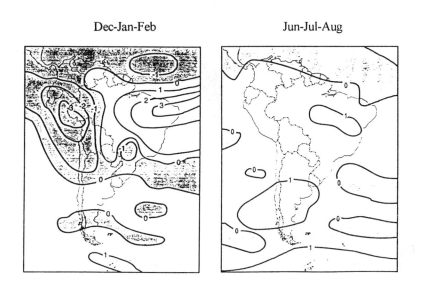

Intercomparison of Global Climate change predictions of rainfall (mm/day) in South America for a doubling C02 of the NCAR and GISS. Mean values for Dec-Jan-Feb and for Jun-Jul-Aug. Stippling indicates decreasing values. (Taken partially from Schlesinger and Mitchell, 1987).

Figure 2.4b   Values for rainfall changes [NCAR Model]

(b)   Produced by socio-economic and cultural quality conditions which contributes
a proliferation of plagues, and human migrations which diffuse the species.
The best example is T. *infestans*, which originated in the Bolivian valleys, with
trophic association with wild guinea-pigs. It was diffused by passive transport
to the south of Ecuador, north of Recife (Brazil) and Patdagonia.

In a wild ecosystem the vector populations are exposed to climatic influences, to
abundance, scarcity or changes in food, and imbalances with predators. Some haemato-
phagus insects can find better conditions when man establishes his home in a transformed
bioma, because they have more refugees, micro-habitats, and permanent food sources.

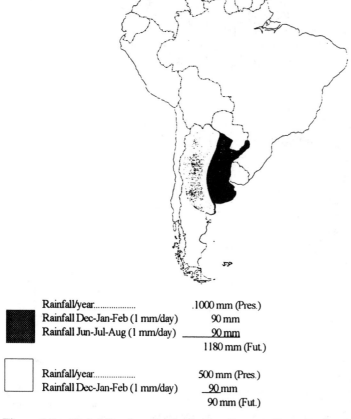

	Rainfall/year...................	.1000 mm (Pres.)
	Rainfall Dec-Jan-Feb (1 mm/day)	90 mm
	Rainfall Jun-Jul-Aug (1 mm/day)	90 mm
		1180 mm (Fut.)
	Rainfall/year...................	500 mm (Pres.)
	Rainfall Dec-Jan-Feb (1 mm/day)	90 mm
		90 mm (Fut.)

**Figure 2.5   Rainfall values for the future climate of Pampa and Chaco [Based in
Giss Predictions]**

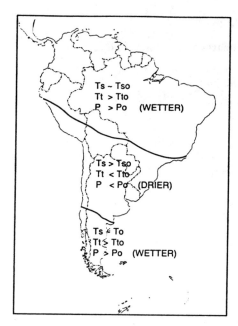

without Amazonic
desforestation

with Amazonic
desforestation

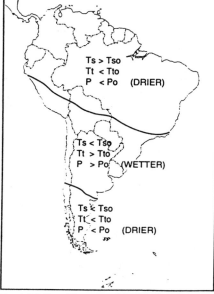

Ts: surface temperature, Tt: tropospheric temperature, P: rainfall. From Hansen et al (1988). The subscript "o" indicates present climate. Symbols and slight decrease or increase.

(Molion, unpublished, 1988 and Burgos, Fuenzalida and Molion, 1991)

Figure 2.6   Molion hypothesis for changes in climatological parameters

Table 2.1

Regional climate changes and their influences on vegetation and vector species.

	Climatic vegetation	Changes A. darling		T. infestans
	Chaco +T -H	thornbush forest	less	more density
Molion hypothesis without Amazonian deforestation	Pampa +T -H	steppe or drier scrub	same	more density
	Patagonia = T + H	grass steppe		do not modify
	Chaco -T +H	prairie mixed forest	less	less density
Molion hypothesis with Amazonian deforestation	Pampa -T +H	same	same	less density
	Patagonia -T -H			less area less density
	Chaco +T+H	dry tropical forest	permanent presence	+ or = density + area
GISS model	Pampa +T+H	savanna	+quantity	+or = density
	Patagonia +T +H	prairie	+permanent	+area +area
NCAR model	Patagonia +T -H	more desert		+area = density

The increases of temperatures would produce a displacement of wild species similar to the isothermal displacement, in conditions of favourable phyto- and zoo-geography for their breeding places.

If temperature increases with more rainfall, the dry tropical forest would extend to the south, and so; the permanent presence of *A. darlingi* would be similar to Bolivia and Brazil in Argentina. In these conditions it can start malaria epidemics in regions with high population density (Table 2.1).

On the other hand, if higher temperatures are followed by diminishing of rainfall (Hypothesis GISS without Amazonian deforestation), the dry forest of Chaco would be transformed into a thornbush forest with worse ecological conditions for *A. darlingi*.

The climatic changes would have no importance to domestic vectors like *T. infestans*, because the internal homeothermia and the dry climates adaptation of species like it is present in the east of Argentina at this time. Only one factor would be important: the increase of population densities in present border areas produced by an increase of days with more than 20°C.

If this increase of temperatures is followed by a diminishing of rainfall (Hypothesis GISS without Amazonian deforestation) the climatic condition would be the best for high density populations of this vector.

References

Aragao, M. B. (1971). "Sobre a dispersao do Triatoma infestans" *Rev. da ociedade Brasileira de Medicina Tropical,* 5 (4): 183-191.

Bejarano, J.F.R. (1959). "Areas Paludicas de la Republica Argentina", *Primeras Jornadas* Entomoepidemilogicas Argentinas, Primera Parte, pp. 275-329.

Bejarano, J.F.R. (1971). "Datos sobre la existencia, biologia y trasmision del paludismo por el *Anopheles (Nyssorhynchus) darlingi* en la Republica Argentina y otros paises de America". *Segundas Jornadas Entomoepidemiologicas Argentinas,* Salta, 2 al 9 de octubre de 1965. Tomo III, pp 289-357.

Blaksley, J. and Carcavallo, R.U. (1968). *La enfermedad de Chagas-Mazza en la Argentina. Estudios entomoepidemiologicos y clinicos,* Buenos Aires, Secretaria de Salud Publica, 140 pp.

Burgos, J.J., Ponche, F.H. and Molion, L.C.B. (1991). "Climate Change Predictions for South America". *Climatic Change,* 18: 223-239.

Canale D.M. and Carcavallo, R.U. (1985). "*Triatoma infestans* (Klug)". In *Factores biologicos y ecologicos de la Enfermedad de Chagas,* 1: 237-250. ECO-OPS/SNCH-MSAS.

Carcavallo, R.U. (1976). "Aspects of the epidemiology of Chagas's disease in Venezuela and Argentina", OPS, *Am. Tryp. Res.,* pp. 347-358.

Carcavallo, R.U. Martinez, A., Canale, D., Becker, D. and Rozemwurzel, H.J., (1988). *Los vectores de la Enfermedad de Chagas en la Republica Argentina.* Premio R.A. Vaccaarezza 1988, Academia Nacional de Medicina, Buenos Aires.

Carcavallo, R.U. and Martinez A. (1968). *Entomoepidemilogia de la Republica Argentina,* Junta de Investigaciones Cientificas de las Fuerzas Armadas Argentinas, Comunicaciones Cientificas No.13, 2 Tomos.

Curto de Casas, S.I. (1983). "Analisis geografico de la endemia Chagas. Indicadores climaticos", *Chagas,* 1, 1:73-79.

Curto de Casas, S.I. (1991). "La distribution geographique de la maladie de Chagas en Argentine", *Revue Belge de Geographie,* 114 annee, 1990, fascicule 4, pp.181-193.

Curto de Casas, S.I. and Boffi, R. (1990). "malaria reinfestation on the Argentine border", I.G.U. Conference on Health and Development, Kingston, Jamaica, *Geojournal,* in print.

Curto de Casas, S.I. and Carcavallo, R.U. (1984). "Limites del triatomismo en la Argentina. Patagonia:, *Chagas*, vol I, no. 4, pp. 35-40.

Hack, W.H. (1955). "Estudios sobre biologia del *Triatoma infestans* (Klug) (Hemiptera, Reduviidae)". Universidad Nacional de Tucuman. Publication No. 709, *Anales del Instituto de Medicina Regional* 4 (2): 125-147.

Hansen, J., Fung, I., Lacis, A., Rind, D., Russell, G., Lebedeff, S., Ruedy, R. and Stone, P. (1987). "Predictions of near-term climate evolution. What can we tell decision-makers now? *Proc. of the First North American Conference on Preparing for Climate Change*. Oct. 27-29. pp 35-44. Washington D.C.

Hansen J., Fung, I., Lacis, A., Rind, D., Russell, G., Lebedeff, S., Ruedy, R., and Stone, P. (1988). "Global Climate Change as Forecast by the Goddard Institute for Space Studies Three Dimensional Model", *J. Geophys. Res.* 93, 9341-9364.

Jorg M.E. (1962). "Influencia de temperatures fijas en periods anuales sobre metamorfosis y fertilidad de Triatoma infestans". *Bol. Chileno de Parasitologia*, 17 (1): 17-19.

Martinez A., and Cichero (1972). *Los vectores de la Enfermedad de Chagas, Lucha conra los mismos en la Argentina*. Direccion Nacional de Promocion y Proteccion de la Salud, Departamento de zoonosis, reservorios y vectores. Ministerio de Bienestar Social, Buenos Aires, Subsecretaria de Salud Publica, Division Imprenta, 56 pp.

Mitchel, C.J. and Darsie, R.F. (1985). "Mosquitoes of Argentina. Part II. Geographic distribution and bibliography". *Mosquito Systematics* 17 (4): 279-360

Schlesinger, M.E. and Mitchell, J.F.B. (1987). "Climate Model Simulations of the Equilibrium Climatic Response to Increased Carbon Dioxide". *Rev. of Geography*. 2 94), 760-798.

Senapa (1991). Servicio Nacional de Paludismo. Unpublished information.

Washington, W.M. and Meehl, G.A. (1983). "General Circulation Model Experiments on the Climatic Effects Due to a Doubling and Quadrupling of Carbon Dioxide Concentration". *J. Geophys. Res.* 88. 6600-6610

Washington, W.M. and Meehl, G.A. (1984). "Seasonal Cycle Experiment on the Climate Sensivity Due to a Doubling CO_2 with an Atmospheric General Circulation Model Coupled to a Simple Mixed-Layed Ocean Model". *J. Geophys. Res.* 89, 9475-9503.

3 Medico-geographical aspects of farming in Africa

S. M. Malkhazova and T. Yu Karimova

Summary

Under the UNEP project, possible medico-geographical problems of agricultural use of lands in Africa were studied. The distribution of over 20 characteristic natural endemic diseases for whose existence biota is a decisive factor was analyzed. Investigation of the impacts of different forms of agricultural production provided an estimate of possible changes in the medico-geographical situation. The results may serve as a basis of measures for the conservation of nature and forecasting the effects of modifications by man on human health.

Introduction

According to expert estimates, to meet the demand of the growing African population, the agricultural produce growth rates towards 1990 should be no less than 4% as against 2% in 1980-1985. (Osaghae, 1987) This prompts an obvious need for a more intensive development of farming, which in its turn may entail substantial changes in the environment. It appears topical to assess the environmental consequences of agricultural production from medico-geographical perspectives. Paradoxical as it may seem, economy-related measures taken in the name of development are often hazardous to the health of the population. (Hunter et al. 1964). Transformation of the foci of diseases existing in natural landscapes, and modification in the forms of contact of the population with them, is a basic medico-geographical problem emerging as a result of changes in ecosystems due to agricultural land use. However, these problems remain insufficiently studied. The present study is aimed at elaboration of approaches to the assessment of the impact of agriculture on the medico-geographical situation (as exemplified by the case study of natural endemic diseases in Africa).

There are two types of epidemic consequences of the anthropogenic changes in natural ecosystems in the process of farming: the immediate ones (short term), appearing in the early stages of the economic development of an area, and the indirect ones (long term), resulting from the agricultural land use.

Early stages of the economic development of the area irrespective of a landscape type always entail growing mosaicism of habitats and extension of the ecotonic community areas, generally accompanied by an intensive circulation of causative agents. More extensive contacts of the population with natural foci in the process of development contribute to increasing epidemic hazard over the area. The influx of substantial non-immune contingents and stepped-up migrations promoting the transmission of an infection favour the epidemic manifestations of foci and a growing disease incidence. Therefore one should expect a certain activization of all the natural endemic diseases at the early area development stages.

The transformation of the ecosystems involved in the agricultural land use produces a variety of impacts on the functioning of foci of natural endemic diseases. In every given case the direction of their evolution depends both on the ecological specificity of co-members of a parasitic system and on the nature of human activity as a form of agricultural land use.

The medico-geographical situation in Africa with regard to the complex of natural endemic diseases and forecasting of its modifications due to the impact of agriculture was estimated using the methods developed by experts of the Institute of Geography of the USSR (now Commonwealth of Independent States (CIS) or Russia Academy of Sciences that we complemented and modified. Early research involved the analysis of geography and ecology of over 20 characteristic natural endemic diseases in Africa, local biota being the decisive factor of their existence. The analysis of their incidence projected against physico-geographical and socio-economical maps resulted in the medico-geographical regionalization of the continent's territory. A total of 22 medico-geographical types of natural endemic diseases complex have been identified in Africa. (Table 3.1)

Findings

The assessment of the epidemic threat involved estimating natural pre-conditions for the existence of diseases within individual medico-geographical types. For this a three point scale was used to estimate the level of the loading of natural pre-conditions of each disease: high (3), moderate (2), low (1). Then the values reflecting the level of the loading of pre-conditions were summarised by all the nosological forms for each medico-geographical type (total index) besides the sum total of the loading of pre-conditions for a group of disease equally involved a diversity (abundance) of characteristic nosological units and the number of diseases exhibiting a high loading of pre-conditions. The following way of recording the total index was used $\frac{A}{B}$ C, where A is a total load ing of pre-conditions,

B is the number of nosological forms and C is the number of nosological forms exhibiting a high loading of pre-conditions.

Table 3.1
Total indices of medico-geographical types of territories

Preconditions		Types of territories				
Natural		I	III	VIII	IX	XV
Related to various forms of farming		$\frac{22}{14}$O	$\frac{37}{16}$g	$\frac{25}{15}$O	$\frac{16}{13}$O	$\frac{3}{3}$O
	with irrigated crop farming		$\frac{40}{16}$11	$\frac{38}{15}$8	$\frac{27}{13}$4	
	with non-irrigated crop farming		$\frac{38}{16}$g	$\frac{28}{15}$1		$\frac{6}{3}$O
	with non irrigated crop farming and livestock breeding		$\frac{40}{17}$g	$\frac{30}{16}$2	$\frac{20}{14}$1	$\frac{7}{4}$O
	with nomadic and semi-nomadic livestock breeding		$\frac{40}{17}$g	$\frac{31}{16}$2	$\frac{22}{14}$2	$\frac{9}{4}$1

The statistical analysis of the total indices obtained provided a class interval and gradations of the loading of pre-conditions for the whole of Africa: under 7 points very low, 7-14 - low, 15-21 - medium, 22-28 - high and over 28 - very high. A cartographic interpretation of the data obtained is featured on the map "Assessment of medico-geographical situation by pre-conditions of diseases". (Fig. 3.1)

The next stage involved the assessment of a possible change in relative loading of natural pre-conditions of all the diseases accompanying the farming land use relying on the available cartographic data on the agricultural impact and ecologic and epidemiologic particularities of co-members of parasitic systems. In each region, its principal forms are determined by specifics of the geographical environment (irrigated crop farming and livestock breeding, non-irrigated crop farming and livestock breeding, nomadic and semi-nomadic cattle breeding). Nosological profiles for every medico-geographical type have been compiled, taking into account the changes mentioned. Fig. 3.2. Total indices characterizing pre-conditions for the diseases to exist against the background of agricul-

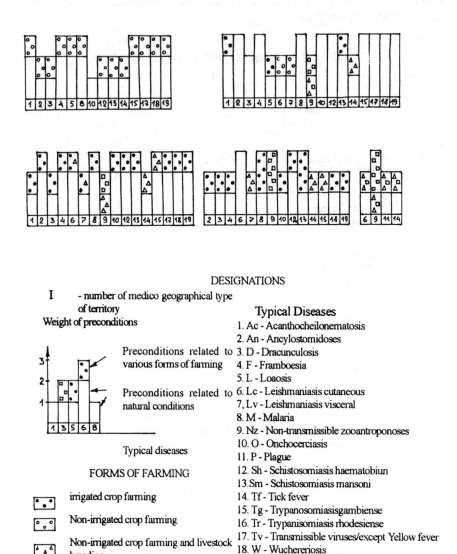

DESIGNATIONS

I   - number of medico geographical type
       of territory

Weight of preconditions

Preconditions related to various forms of farming

Preconditions related to natural conditions

Typical diseases

FORMS OF FARMING

irrigated crop farming

Non-irrigated crop farming

Non-irrigated crop farming and livestock breeding

nomadic and semi-nomadic livestock breeding

Typical Diseases

1. Ac - Acanthocheilonematosis
2. An - Ancylostomidoses
3. D - Dracunculosis
4. F - Framboesia
5. L - Loaosis
6. Lc - Leishmaniasis cutaneous
7, Lv - Leishmaniasis visceral
8. M - Malaria
9. Nz - Non-transmissible zooantroponoses
10. O - Onchocerciasis
11. P - Plague
12. Sh - Schistosomiasis haematobiun
13.Sm - Schistosomiasis mansoni
14. Tf - Tick fever
15. Tg - Trypanosomiasisgambiense
16. Tr - Trypanisomiasis rhodesiense
17. Tv - Transmissible viruses/except Yellow fever
18. W - Wuchereriosis
19. Yf - Yellow fever

Figure 3.1   Nosological profiles

36

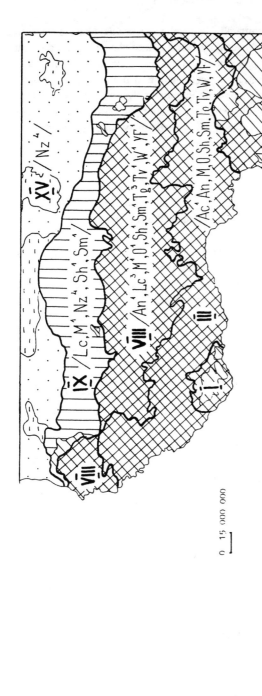

Figure 3.2 Forecasting of medico geographical consequences of farming [West Africa, frag.]

F - diseases revealing a high loading
  weight of natural preconditions

M high preconditions weight diseases in
  various forms of farming: 1. irrigated
  crop farming, 2. non-irrigated crop
  farming, 3. non-irrigated crop farming
  and livestock breeding, 4. nomadic and
  semi-nomadic livestock breeding

Weight of preconditions

very low

low
moderate

high

very high

0 15 000 000

37

tural production have also been estimated. A nosological profile features data on characteristic nosoforms spread over the territory. Besides, it contains forecasts on what is going to occur to relative loadings of pre-conditions for the above diseases as the territory is being economically developed, i.e. as natural ecosystems turn into anthropogenic ones. Analyzed materials show that growing economic activity involves a build-up in relative loadings of pre-conditions for diseases to exist over a major part of the continent. The data thus obtained served as a base for compiling a summary map "Forecasting of medico-geographical consequences of farming" (Fig. 3.2).

Results and discussion

Its analysis indicates that the medico-geographical situation with respect to a possible development of farming in Africa is likely to undergo the following transformations. There is a very high level of relative loadings of pre-conditions for diseases in Central Africa within the area between latitude 10° North and latitude 10° South up to longitude 38° East where up to 17 various nosoforms can possibly exist in different natural farming areas. Especially great is the threat of malaria, trypanosomiasis gambiense, loaosis, wuche-rereiosis, transmissible viruses and also framboesia and yellow fever (north of latitude 6° South). North of latitude 8° North the above disease are joined by schistosomiases, onchoceraciasis, visceral and cutaneous leishmaniases, ancylostomidoses, acanthocheilonematosis and non-transmissible zoonoses (in livestock breeding development areas). South of latitude 6° South, there is a high incidence of schistosomiases and ancylostomidoses besides general diseases. Over the remaining part of Africa areas of very high loadings of pre-conditions are to be encountered locally. These are the regions of the Ethiopian plateau, the upper and middle Zambezi river and the upper Nile river.

The areas of high relative loadings of pre-conditions are primarily located to the south east of the preceding area. 14 diseases can spread here. Particularly hazardous are malaria, schistosomiases, wuchereriosis, trypanosomiasis rhodesiense, ancylostomidoses, transmissible viruses, loaosis and the plague. Over the rest of Africa there are high relative loadings of pre-conditions in the valley of river Nile, in the basins of the rivers Senegal, Niger, Zambezi, Jubba and Webi-Shebeli, on the Mediterranean coast and in the central part of the island of Madagascar.

Areas with moderate relative pre-conditions loadings take up the rest of the territory between latitude 15° North and 20° South in the West and 25° South in the East. Up to 12 diseases can possibly persist here. In the North, there is a substantial incidence of malaria, schistosomiasis haematobium, cutaneous and visceral leishmaniases, ancylostomidoses, wuchereriosis and non-transmissible zoonoses. In the south there are the most favourable conditions for the transmission of malaria, schistosomiases, ancylostomidoses, transmissible viruses and non-transmissible zoonoses. Small areas exhibiting moderate pre-conditions loadings are located in the basin of the Orange river, in oases, on the west and east coast of the island Madagascar.

The rest of the continent with the exception of the far south is constituted by the areas having a low loading of pre-conditions. Up to 8 nosoforms are reported there, with a high incidence rate of non-transmissible zoonoses and the plague in the south.

In the extreme south of Africa there are regions exhibiting an extremely low loading of pre-conditions 5-6 diseases are reported to persist but environmental conditions are unfavourable for the intensive circulation of causative agents and pre-condition loadings for nosoform infections are low.

Conclusion

Summing up a tentative forecasting of modifications in the medico-geographical situation in Africa occurring due to the impact of farming, it is necessary to emphasize that in the absence of a special prevention and sanitation drive the situation might be aggravated. Therefore there is a pressing need for the development of medico-geographical maps containing estimates and forecasts for individual regions to be developed. The findings of investigations in the domain of medical geography should become the cornerstone for the comprehensive planning of agricultural use of a territory.

References

Environment and human health - Moscow, *Nauka*. (1979). 214 p. (in Rus.)

Hunter, D.M., Ray. I., and Scott, D. (1984). Development of water resources and health of the population. *World Health Forum.* 79-85. (in Rus.)

Osaghae, E.E. (1987). The African food crisis and the crisis of development in Africa. A theoretical exploration. *Afr. Quarterly*, 34-51.

Voronou, A.G., Malkhazova, S.M., Komarova, L.U. (1982). Assessment of medico-geographical situation over the territory of the Median region and forecasting of possible changes due to water diversion. *Proceeding of the Academy of Sciences of the USSR, Geographical Series.* Moscow. 2: 30-39. (in Rus.)

4 Effects of rural development on the decline of endemic disease incidence in Se-deficient areas in China

Tan Jian'an, Zhu Wenya, Li Ribang, Wang Wuyi and Hou Shaofan

Summary

It has been proved that Keshan disease and Kaschin-Beck disease, two endemic diseases occurring in China, are associated with selenium (Se) deficiency. They usually occur in the areas where the selenium in geo-ecosystems is always low; and we could control them by giving selenium supplement to the people in the affected area. Since the 1980s, the incidence rates of the two diseases have obviously decreased. The present paper mainly deals with the causal reasons for the decline incidence of the two diseases. An investigation in the disease belt has been conducted over recent years. Results show that since the earlier studies of the 1970's, no apparent changes have been found in Se content in the soil cereals; however, the level of Se in human hair has elevated. It means that the raising of selenium levels in the hair, which usually indicates an improvement in Se intake, results mainly from the economic development in the affected area, partly or locally from the direct Se supplementation to the population in affected areas, and very little from the change of Se content in soils and cereals.

Introduction

Two endemic diseases, Keshan disease (KSD) and Kaschin-Beck disease (KBD), have been observed in China, in Transbaikalia of the former USSR and in the northern part of Korea. Keshan disease is an endemic cardiomyopathy in human beings. Its pathological changes mainly involve the myocardium. Serious myocardial degeneration, necrosis and scar formation are indicated. The principal clinical manifestations are acute and chronic cardiac insufficiency, acute cardiac failure, heart enlargement, gallop rhythm, arrhythmia and electrocardiogram changes. Kaschin-Beck disease is an endemic osteoarthropathy. Major changes are chondral degeneration and chondron necrosis, as well as repair process following necrosis mainly in joint cartilage and the epiphyseal plate of the four limbs.

T. Jian'an, Z. Wenya, L. Ribang, W. Wuyi and H. Shaofan

The main clinical symptoms are painful, thickened and deformed joints of the four limbs, with atrophied muscles and difficulty in stretching and bending limbs. In severe cases, fingers, toes and limbs may shorten and result in deformation.

The pathogeny of the two diseases was unknown for a long time. A variety of pathogenic hypotheses, including biological and non-biological forms were suggested, but no quite satisfactory evidence to support the hypotheses was available. No break-through in pathogenic exploration of both diseases was made until the 1970's. Since then there have been two important findings in the exploration, drawing an extensive and strong interest of the researchers at home and abroad. They are (1) The two diseases are always situated in a low selenium eco-environment which geographically forms a low selenium belt coinciding with the distribution of the two diseases (EGAS 1974, 1976, 1979, Tan Jian'an et al 1989), (2) Selenium use in prevention and treatment of the two diseases achieved a great success (Keshan disease Research Group, 1979, Li Chenzhen 1979). Then it was proved that these diseases were closely related to a selenium-deficient environment and in the meantime the direct relationship between selenium deficiency and human health was first identified.

Since the 1980s, the incidence of the diseases has decreased to a varied degree, and in some places has even been basically controlled. However, the reason for the decrease of the disease incidence was not clear; the relation of selenium deficiency to the two diseases came under suspicion. The present paper mainly studied this problem. Through our recent investigation of late years, we have made it relatively clear. It has been found that the decline of incidence of the diseases is associated with the elevation of the Se intake level in population from the affected areas. Raising of the Se intake is caused by polyfactors. But the rapid development of the rural economy and improvement of living standard, due to the reform and open policy, have played an important role. It means that fresh progress has been made in the course of the pathogenic study on the two diseases.

Principal characteristics of geographical epidemiology

In China Keshan disease is distributed in 309 counties of 15 provinces and autonomous regions including Heilongjiang, Jilin, Lianoning, Nei Monggol (Inner Mongolia), Hebei, Shangdong, Shanxi, Henan, Shaanxi, Gansu, Sichuan, Yunan, Xizang (Tibet), Hubei and Guizhou; and the Kaschin-Beck disease is recorded in 303 counties of 15 provinces, autonomous regions, and municipalities including Heilongjiang, Jilin, Lianoing, Nei Monggol, Hebei, Beijing (a suburban county), Shangdong, Shanxi, Henan, Shaanxi, Gansu, Qinghai, Sichuan, Xizang and Taiwan. From this it can be seen that the distribution of the two diseases is quite similar (Fig. 4.1). They occur commonly in most of the provinces afore-mentioned, geographically forming a disease belt stretching from the north east to the south west.

The distribution of the Keshan disease and Kaschin-Beck disease are very orderly, and closely relates to the geographical environment. They are mainly distributed in the broad transitional belt, running from NE to SW, with the temperate (or warm temperate) forest and forest-steppe soils as the axis, while the typical steppe and desert zones to the north-west and the typical yellow and red earth zones to the south-east are generally disease-free. Therefore, three belts can be distinctly distinguished. The disease-affected belt is situated in the middle, with both the north-west and to the south-east being disease-free belts. Furthermore, within the disease belt these two diseases always occur in the mountainous and hilly land and valley flats, while the large alluvial plains are usually free of these diseases. The landscapes of the disease-affected areas mainly belong to three types: temperate forest and forest-steppe landscape, eroded loess upland landscape and purlish soil landscape.

As regards the vulnerability of population group to the diseases, the people from agricultural households in the disease belt, consuming locally-produced grain as the staple food stuff, are most susceptible. Kaschin-Beck disease can be seen in children or teenagers; the prevalence rate may be ever 50% in children under ten in some seriously affected villages. No apparent differences in disease occurrence have been found between the sexes. As to Kashan disease, in North China, children under ten years of age and women of child-bearing age used to be the main victims in earlier years. Later, the proportion of child victims has risen. However, in south west China, children under ten years of age have always been the chief victims. Based on a systematic statistics collected from 1959-1982, the average annual incidence rate for the acute and subacute forms of the disease was 9.3 cases per 100,000 persons on the whole affected areas of the country, while the prevalence rate for the chronic form mostly ranged from 1.0-150.0 cases per 100,000 persons by county. Up to 1990 the incidence rate for acute and subacute forms fell to 0.33 cases per 100,000 persons.

Association of selenium deficiency in the geo-ecosystem to endemic diseases

It has been shown that selenium deficiency is associated with the diseases, KSD and KBD. We have measured selenium concentration in geo-ecosystematic substances, such as rock, soil, plant, herbage, grain, animal and human hair, even some issues of man collected from different places within the country (Fig. 4.2).

As our early studies have reported (Tan Jian'an *et al*, 1984; EGAS 1979, 1981, 1982, 1984), the geographical distribution laws of selenium were found as follows,

(1)   Low Se environments occur mainly in and near temperate forest and forest-steppe landscapes as an axis in China; while sufficient selenium environments are situated in tropical, subtropical, desert and steppe areas (Fig. 4.2).

(2)   In young soil or landscape, selenium of the parent material is a very important factor controlling the distribution of this element in geographical ecosystems.

43

T. Jian'an, Z. Wenya, L. Ribang, W. Wuyi and H. Shaofan

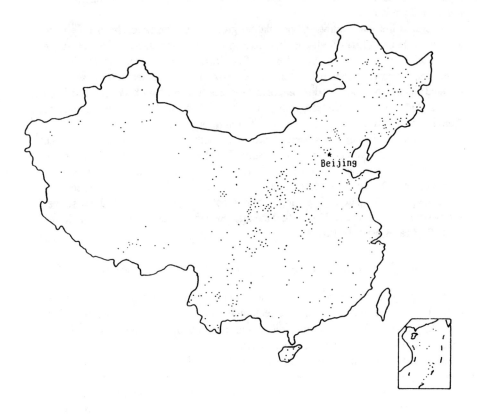

Figure 4.1   Sample collection sites, 1977, in China

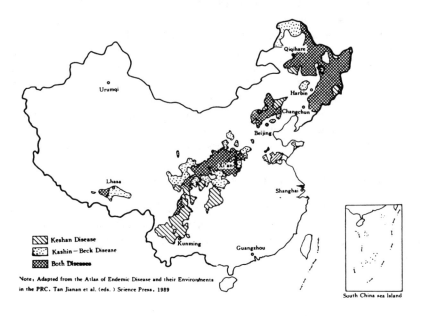

Figure 4.2   Distribution of keshan disease and kaschin beck disease in China

(3)   The distribution of the low-Se environment is also associated with the change of the vertical geographical zone in some high mountainous areas, such as in south west China.

(4)   There is a relatively high selenium level in some large accumulation plains. Finally, the four distribution laws of selenium concluded above basically dominated the patterns and structures of selenium distribution in geo-ecosystems in China, as seen in Fig. 4.3.

Importantly it was discovered that Keshan disease and Kaschin-Beck disease always appeared in low selenium environments. The research results were summarized in Table 4.1. So in geographical terms the distribution of KSD and KBD usually coincides well with that of a low selenium environment. All of these points enable us to formulate a series of Se-threshold values for distinguishing the disease area from a non-disease area. For example, the threshold value of soil total Se is 0.125-0.175 ppm. Soil water-soluble Se, 0.003 ppm; Food grain Se, 0.02ppm, hair Se, 0.20ppm.

Another persuasive fact is that a lot of work on supplementation of selenium in different forms to control incidence of the disease have achieved a great success. The present paper mainly deals with the relationship of incidence rate decrease to rural development.

Influence of rural development on Se intake level and disease incidence

In studying the relation of selenium with KSD and KBD we have found that the rural economic development and raising of living standards in affected areas play a beneficial role to increasing the Se intake of human body and then controlling the two diseases.

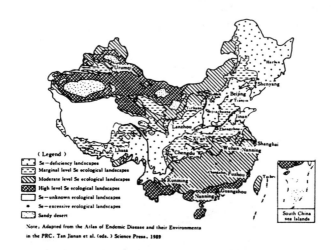

Figure 4.3   Selenium ecological landscape map of China

46

Table 4.1
Relation of selenium in geo-ecosystem subsistances with the diseases and landscape types (ppm)

Landscape type	Disease	Soil	Maize	Rice	Wheat	Hair
Temperate desert and steppe	No	0.19	0.049	0.087	0.106	0.329
(NW sufficient Se belt)		(29)	(69)	(25)	(15)	(371)
Temperate forest and forest		0.13	0.015	0.022	0.021	0.129
Steppe (Middle low Se belt)		(80)	(230)	(120)	(272)	(1412)
Among	KSD	KBD	0.17	0.014	0.012	0.140
		(5)	(8)	(5)	(56)	
	KSD	0.09	0.013	0.011	0.018	0.085
		(16)	(55)	(51)	(72)	(851)
	KBD	0.09	0.009	-	0.011	,
		(15)	(3)		(27)	,
	No	0.09	0.019	0.031	0.026	0.187
		(29)	(91)	(64)	(117)	(597)
Tropical and subtropical forest	No	0.23	0.053	0.062	0.056	0.376
(Se sufficient Se belt)		(77)	(16)	(256)	(71)	(245)

Note: The Digits in Brackets Are Numbers of Samples

Since the 1980s, the incidence of the two diseases have extensively appeared apparently to decrease. A new problem has arisen: What is the reason for the decrease of the two diseases? Over recent years our research group, in collaboration with other 9 institutions, has dealt with the problem to find out the origin causing this decrease of incidence. The sampling side for geo-ecosystem substances including rock, soil, food grains, drinking water, human hair etc. are scattered over all the provinces with endemic disease (Fig.4. 4). Selenium contents in different samples from the entire disease belt have been determined, and compared with the measured data of selenium in soil, food grains and hair earlier collected from there. The results are shown in Tables 4.2- 4.3.

From Table 4.2, we were able to find that selenium concentrations in soil, corn, rice and wheat in the 1980s have shown quite small changes, compared with those of the 1970s. However, the selenium concentration of hair in the disease areas obviously increased, always being over or near the hair threshold value of 0.2ppm, which separates the disease area from the non-disease area. Table 4.3 showed that in 8 of 16 provinces with diseases, the Se content of hair in disease areas has been over or near the threshold value 0.200ppm. It indicated that raised hair selenium means an improvement in Se intake, because Se content level in hair usually is one of the suitable indicators for the Se level in the whole body. So the research work made it clear that since the 1980s, the incidence of the two diseases was closely related with the increase of Se intake in the population of affected area. Then new evidence supportive of the association of the diseases with Se deficiency was achieved.

For the reason causing the elevation of hair Se level in affected areas, there are five points, as follows:

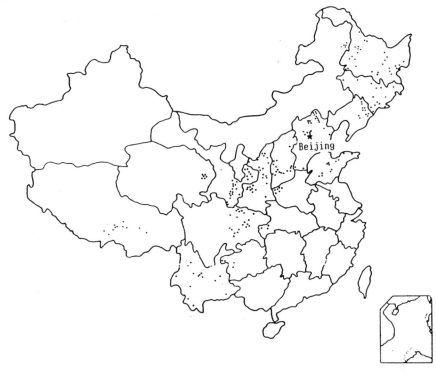

Figure 4.4   **Sampling sites in keshan disease survey**

Table 4.2

Comparison of Se in food grain and hair of the 1970s with that of the 1980s (ppm)

Area	NW Sufficient Se Belt	Middle Low Se Belt		SE Sufficient Se Belt
Year	1970s	1970s	1980s	1970s
Disease	No	KSD, KBD	KSD, KBD	No
Maize (corn)	0.049 + 0.031	0.013 + 0.006	0.010 + 0.009	0.053 + 0.028
	(69)	(157)	(90)	(16)
Rice	0.087 + 0.046	0.014 + 0.007	0.015 + 0.011	0.064 + 0.031
	(25)	(115)	(31)	(256)
Wheat	0.106 + 0.092	0.014 + 0.008	0.013 + 0.010	0.052 + 0.026
	(157)	(47)	(96)	(71)
Hair	0.389	0.085 + 0.032	0.192 + 0.096	0.387
	(371)	(815)	(144)	(245)
Soil	0.19	0.13	0.128	0.23
	(79)	(80)	(123)	(77)

Note: The Digits in Brackets are Numbers of Sample.

Table 4.3

Hair selenium content in disease area from the provinces with disease in the 1980s (ppm)

Province		Se Content
Gansu		0.187 + 0.157 (176)
Heilongjia		0.206 + 0.055(23)
Liaoning		0.255 + 0.002(2)
Jilin		0.147 + 0.047 (31)
Hebei		0.208 + 0.083 (108)
Henan		0.163 + 0.073 (51)
Shaanxi	1970s	0.096 + 0.012 (14)
	1980s	0.234 + 0.081 (14)
Shanxi		0.193 + 0.096 (104)
Shandong		0.151 + 0.047 (74)
Nei Monggol		0.060 + 0.024 (18)
Sichuan		0.129 + 0.060 (109)
Yunnan		0.131 + 0.051 (7)
Guizhou		0.236 + 0.021 (2)
Qinghai		0.106 + 0.016 (14)
Xizang 0		.215 + 0.109 (10)

Note: The Digits in Parenthesis are Numbers of Samples

(1) The economic development in rural areas under the reform and open policy enable the people affected to improve their living standard, and then the Se ecological cycle of the affected area.

(2) Since the middle of 1970s, the measures of Se supplementation for controlling the diseases have been extensively spread in affected areas, especially in some provinces such as Heilongjiang, Shaanxi, Hebei etc.

(3) The growing structure of crops and dietary composition are changed greatly. In the past years, maize (corn) poor in Se usually constitutes the staple food grain of the local rural residents in disease areas. At the present time the proportion of corn to the diet as a whole was apparently decreased. However, the proportion of wheat was correspondingly greatly increased (Table 4.4). Usually wheat is relatively rich in selenium, compared with maize

(4) The food grains from the non-disease regions, which used to be more rich in Se than that from disease area itself, were imported into the affected area. Then the Se cycle level in the affected area could be raised through the food grain exchange between the disease and non-disease regions. All of these indicated that the control of KSD and KBD could be achieved through raising the Se ecological cycle by means of economic-ecological measures.

Table 4.4

The relation of staple grain composition in the diet with KSD incidence in Huanglong county, Shaanxi province by survey of three villages

Years	Wheat Rate	Maize (Corn) Rate	Soybean and Others	Incidence
	%	%	%	(cases)
1965-1966	5.6	89.2	5.2	1042
1967-1972	10.2	82.7	7.1	362
1973-1979	31.8	59.1	9.1	112
1980-1982	80.8	7.3	11.9	0
1983-1988	79.6	13.4	10.0	0

From the Joint Group for KSD and Environmental Se 1991.

Conclusion

Keshan disease and Kaschin-Beck disease are two endemic diseases which occur in Se-deficient area. The present paper has further established that the incidence of the two diseases could be influenced by change in the Se intake and the rural development could affect the Se intake and then the incidence of the two diseases. So we could control the disease through the rural development and improvement of Se ecocycle.

References

EGAS (The Group of Environment and Endemic Diseases, Institute of Geography, Chinese Academy of Sciences) 1976. *The environmental etiology of Keshan disease.* unpublished Research Report

EGAS 1979. The Keshan disease in China, A study of the geographical epidemiology. *Acta Geographia Sinica*, 34, 85-103.

EGAS 1981. The relationship between the distribution of Keshan disease and the Selenium Content of Food Grain as a Factor of Chemical Geographical Environment. *Acta Geographia Sinica*, 36, 369-376.

EGAS 1982. Geographical distribution of selenium content in human hair in Keshan disease and nondisease zones in China. *Acta Geographia Sinica*, 37, 136-143.

EGAS 1984. Geographical Distribution of Selenium Content in the Top Soils in China and its Association with Selenium Responsive Disease in Man and Animals. *Geographical Research* 3, 39-47.

Li Chongzheng 1979. 'Effect of Se and Vitamin on 224 X-ray Cases for Kaschin-Beck disease and exploration of Disease Causation.' *National Medical Journal of China* 59(3)

Keshan disease Research Group of the Chinese, AMS, 1979. 'Observation on the effect of sodium selenite in prevention of Keshan disease.' *Chinese Med. J. 92*, 471.

Tan Jian'an 1982a. The Keshan disease in China, a Study of Ecological Chemicogeography. *The National Geographical Journal of India.* 28, 15-18.

Tan Jian'an *et al.* 1982b, The Retention of Keshan disease to Natural Environment and the Background of Selenium Nutrition. *Acta Nutrimenta* 4, 175-181.

Tan Jian'an 1984. Setenium Ecological Chemicogeography and Endemic Keshan disease and Kasch-Beck disease in China. *Selenium in Biology and Medicine*, edited by Van Nostrand Reinhold Company, New York (1987) 859-876.

Tan Jian'an et al. 1985. The characteristics of Geographical Epidemiology for Kaschin-Back Disease in China and its Pathogenicity. *Scienta Geographia Sinica*, 5 1-8.

Tan Jian'an et al. 1988, Selenium in Environment and Kaschin-Beck Disease. *Chinese Journal of Geochemistry*, 7, 373-380.

Tan Jian'an 1990. The Influence of Selenium Deficiency in Environment on Human Health in North east China. Excess and Deficiency of Trace Elements in Relation to Human and Animal Health in Arctic and Subarctic Regions, edited by J. Lag. NASL, 90-108.

The Joint Group of Keshan disease and Environmental Selenium 1991. New Progress in the Causal Association of Keshan disease with Environmental Selenium in China. *Chinese Journal of Endemiology*, 10(5) 269-274.

5 Water supply and guinea worm disease in O.C.C.G.E. countries: Geographical study of transmission and diffusion

Gustave Yameogo

Summary

Dracunculiasis (guinea worm disease) is a major health problem in West Africa in general, and particularly in O.C.C.G.E. countries. This disease is very common in poor agricultural regions of these developing countries. Because dracunculiasis is a disabilitating condition, it disorganises and lowers agricultural production. The only source of infection is dirty water containing microfilariae-infested cyclops. Man constitutes the only reservoir of adult parasites. Geographical studies, using a spatial approach, and studying the environment-society relationship, can lead to a better understanding of the transmission and of the spread of the disease. This communication does not aim to present results, but only to propose a geographical methodology.

Introduction

On the top of other problems that African developing countries are facing, water quality and water availability adds to the burden of African populations. As a matter of fact, in these countries, water is considered to be the cause of many diseases of viral, bacterial or parasitic origin. Problems relating to this essential resource, are more crucial in the rural area, where the majority of developing countries' population live.

In 1981, the objectives of the United Nations decade of drinking water and water supply (1981-1990) were:

- to provide access to a clean water supply for every one.
- health education in order to increase the awareness of the need for a clean water supply.

In spite of the efforts put in by populations and other agencies, these objectives have not been reached yet. In most developing countries, rural populations still require a clean water supply.

Guinea worm disease or dracunculiasis has only one cause: drinking water containing cyclops infected with guinea worm microfilariae. The preferential site of those crustaceans are ponds. After ingestion by a human being, microfilariae become adult worms that move under the skin until they reach a point where they will come out and form an ulcer; creating then a potential entry for tetanus. Emerging adult worms release microfilariae when infected person with an ulcer enters a pond. These microfilariae will then infect other cyclops completing the parasitic cycle.

Human behaviour is involved at two essential levels of the guinea worm cycle: Firstly, entering a pond with guinea worm ulcers introduces Dracunculus medinensis in the cyclops breeding site; secondly drinking dirty water containing infested cyclops allows human infestation.

However, the guinea worm parasitic cycle is theoretically easy to break, since drinking water is the only source of contamination and man the only reservoir of adult parasites. For those two reasons, the 44th World Health Assembly passed a resolution (WHA 44.5) which aims to eradicate guinea worm disease by the year 1995.

Guinea worm disease is present in many countries throughout the world. (West Africa, Asia, Pakistan and West India). Annual incidence is estimated to be 5 to 10 millions cases and 140 million persons are exposed to the parasite world-wide. Incidence is highest in the 10 to 50 years old age group. Guinea worm is endemic in West Africa, where its distribution stretches along Sahelian countries. Transmission is seasonal but may occur during rainy or dry season according to local ecology.

The study zone

The O.C.C.G.E. zone is situated in West Africa between latitude 5° and 25° North. The endemic area is approximately located between lattitude 5° and 16° North and therefore include:

(1) Sub-equatorial area (South of latitude 9° North, almost equatorial area: South of Ivory Coast, of Benin and Togo).
   There is no dry season, because there is no three month period with less than 50 mm rainfall monthly).

(2) Tropical area (between latitude 9° and 14° North: Senegal, Southern Mali, Central and South Burkina-Faso and South Niger).
   Most of O.C.C.G.E. countries territories are included in this zone. Total rainfall fluctuates between 1500 mm in the South and 500 mm in the North. Within this tropical area, three different regions can be distinguished

   – A southern region (rainfall between 1000 and 1500 mm for six months or more)

   – A northern region (rainfall between 600 and 1000mm in less than 5 months).

- Sahelian region (rainfall between 200mm and 600mm in less than three months

(3) Arid area, where the air is dry and where scanty rains do not exceed 200 mm a year.

Table 5.1 shows the variation in guinea worm disease incidence according to the notification system.

Table 5.1
Situation of guinea worm disease in O.C.C.G.E. countries: dracunculiasis cases reported, 1986-1990

Country	1986	1987	1988	1989	1990
Benin	-	400	33,962	7,172	37,414*
B. Faso	2,558	1,957	1,266	45,004	42,487
I. Coast	1,177	1,272	1,370	1,555	1,360
Mali	5,640	435	564	111	884
Mauritania	-	227	608	447	8,036*
Niger	669	-	228	-	
Senegal	128	132	138	-	38
Togo	1,325	-	178	2,749	3,042

Source: Reievé épidémilogiue hebdomadaire, 1991.

*Data from national surveys or active reporting campaigns. Other incidences come from passive reporting systems.

In O.C.C.G.E. countries, active reporting surveys have been undertaken or are at the point of being undertaken. These projects have been funded by UNICEF and carried out by Health departments in O.C.C.G.E.

Economic impact

Economic impact of dracunculiasis is considerable. It disorganizes and lowers agricultural production. As a matter of fact, working active adults represent the high risk group for guinea worm disease. Moreover, the guinea worm transmission season frequently overlaps with the rainy season, which is the time when people are active doing agricultural work. Field studies have been carried out in South West Burkina Faso (Guiguemde, et al., 1986) Some of the main results are summarised on Table 5.2.

According to this study, in the villages investigated, guinea worm incidence peaks during the rainy season, which is the period of agricultural work. Ninety percent of guinea worm episodes exactly occur when peasants should be out working in the fields.

Moreover, the burden of secondary disability is high and paralyses these activities (Fig. 5.1)

These results demonstrate the need to study the transmission and the distribution of this disease according to place and space, so that prevention methods adaptable to different contexts can be found.

Table 5.2

Mean length of total-disability studied in 433 persons in 3 villages of Burkina Faso

	total number of disability days	number of persons affected	mean number of disability days	total number of disability days	number of persons affected	mean number of disability days
	All patients			Patients 16-50 years old		
village 1	2912	152	19,16	1695	62	27,34
village 2	824	114	7 23	421	54	7,80
village 3	3860	167	23,11	2332	71	32,85
Total	7596	433	17,54	4448	187	23,79

*Total disability preventing all agricultural works

Source: TR Guiguemde et al., 1986.

Geographical approach of transmission and diffusion

It is now possible to compare data from one country with data from another, allowing a good geographical approach because identical survey methods are being used in these countries. Results of national active detection surveys now give interesting information to geographers:

They help to resolve the problem of missing data. As a matter of fact, "missing or wrong information do not allow any proper geographical approach" (Gerard, 1988)

These data allow geographers to describe the distribution of guinea worm disease by the means of a map. This tool is very useful for raising questions and for trying to answer some of them.

The aim of this work is different from that of medical sciences. Space is the point of interest, as areas of different risk must be identified and an explanation must be found. Studying the disease is an alibi to do geography.

Geography studies the differences in dracunculiasis expression in different groups, and tries to explain why things are where they are.

Dracunculiasis in rural areas of developing countries is a disease essentially linked to the water supply. The study zone is characterized by a diversity in climate and a diversity in annual rainfall. This diversity explains the differences of water availability that we observe, because most of the water sources come from rainfall. Moreover, social differences between ethnic groups introduces another cause of variability, as different behaviours in water use explains different epidemiological patterns. But, although the endemic zone of dracunculiasis in Africa is known today, spatial variations in our study zone are not always apparent and/or understood. Intervention strategies may then not be adapted to different geographic patterns.

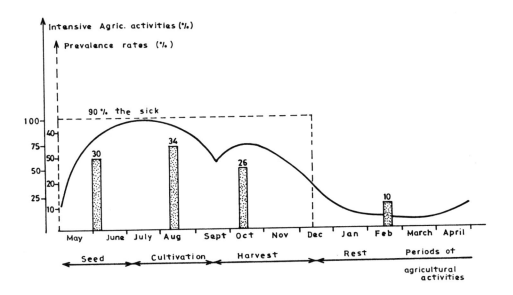

Figure 5.1 **Prevalence of guinea worm disease according to intensity of agricultural work in south-west Burkina-Faso.**

Source: T.R. Guiguemde et al. 1986

Conclusion

This communication seeks not to present the results of a completed study, but rather to propose a geographical approach that could contribute to a better knowledge of particular health problems in Africa.

The aim of this study is to:
- Describe the spatial distribution of dracunculiasis in the O.C.C.G.E. states;
- identify the risk factors for guinea worm disease by means of an analysis of the relationship between people and water, according to the geographical and sociological context;
- to collect useful information for national eradication programs.

The specific points of the geographical approach are to
- use the data from the national active reporting surveys, in order to draw a map of the distribution of dracunculiasis in O.C.C.G.E. states; to classify the typical villages according to climatic context, incidence and sociological background in order to carry out field studies. The identification of the water sources used by the population is very important. The geographical approach shall use multivariate analysis in order to yield information about situations and behaviours that are risk factors for guinea worm disease. The conclusion of the study would help to adapt national eradication programs to specific sociological and geographical contexts.

References

Gbary, A.R., Guiguemde, T.R. and Steib (1986). Cycle de Dévelopment et modalité de la transmission, faciès épidemiologiques. Etudes Médicales, 2:67-76.

Gerard, R. (1988). Paysages et milieux épidémiologiques dans l'espace iviroburkinabè, Mémoire du Centre d'Etudes de Géographie Tropicale, Edition dn CNRS, Paris.

Guiguemde, T.R. Orivel, F., Gbary, A.R. and Ouedraogo, J.B. (1986). Etúdes Medicales, No. 3.

Reievé epidémiologique hebdomadaire (1991).

Part II
URBANIZATION AND HEALTH

Introduction

Rais Akhtar

There has been a tremendous growth in the process of urbanization since the 1950s - much greater than in the whole history of human civilization. This has led to the growing awareness about the impact of urbanization on human health. Urbanization is a complex process of social change affecting the entire nations of the world. The various technological advances of the world have brought a lot of pressure on the urban environment and this has been accentuated by the rural-urban and urban-urban migration. The continued urbanization of most cities of the world have had beneficial and deleterious effects so much so that most of the rapid and sometimes radical changes in the socio-economic and physical transformation of man have been linked to urbanization. A major element of concern in urbanization from time immemorial has been the health of the populace. Most of the earliest legislations about the physical layout of towns and cities were prompted by the desire to enforce sanitary conditions or laws.

This is because many health problems in both the developed and the developing world were and are still related to bad housing conditions, poverty and unemployment, environmental pollution (water, air) and a stressful way of life of urban dwellers. It is a matter of concern that despite the technological gain in health research, the developing countries continue to suffer from poverty and insanitary environment induced diseases and also from the sophisticated diseases of the developed nations such as heart diseases, cancer, drug-abuse, STDs and now AIDS. While these problems continue to assume new dimensions and increasing complexity, various methods have been suggested and indeed experimented to deal with these urbanisation induced health problems.

This section of the book looks at the incidences of these problems in different areas of the world, from different perspectives and by different professionals. The first paper in this section by Layi Egunjobi assumed that there is a relationship between the level of urban sanitary and health conditions and the extent of urban planning activities. This relationship, if it exists, measures the quality of the urban environment (in largest metropolis (in areal extent) in Africa, using selected indicators. Rais Akhtar was of the opinion that the presence of medical facilities is necessary but not sufficient to ensure adequate health conditions without the presence of other vital social services. Research results from the environmental perception surveys in Srinagar, India show that individual and community perception coincided in the assessment of health hazards of the community. The Indian survey results were also ably confirmed in Colombo, Sri Lanka as shown in a survey of health issues in a low income settlement by Wanasinghe.

The last two papers in this section are on Nigeria and reflect the views of earlier researches in another context. For instance Agbola and Akinbamijo assessed the epidemiological contribution/conditions as applied to the housing types in an ancient city of Abeokuta in South Western Nigeria. This was done by examining the role of tenement characteristics on the health of urban dwellers in the city and the study confirm that housing types and tenure affect the health condition of residents. Lastly, Alokan presents a holistic appraisal of the environmental and health consequences of transportation on the populace. Emphasis are on road accidents, air and noise pollution.

This overview shows the wide latitude of the research focus and interest of researchers and indeed of that of environmental health. Discussions and research findings have ranged from localized examples to national treatment or differing environmental issues with an equally large means for improved performances and urban life styles.

6 Urban environmental health and physical planning

Layi Egunjobi

Summary

Attention has long been drawn to the generally intolerable urban environmental living conditions in the developing countries. These are evidenced by overcrowding, lack of potable water supply, inadequate drains, absence and/or inadequate waste disposal facilities, air pollution etc. all of which are causal factors for various diseases.

The objective of this study is to assess the quality of the Ibadan urban environment in terms of selected indicators and relate these to the degree of urban planning activities in various neighbourhoods of the city.

The basic assumption of the study is that there is a relationship between the level of urban sanitary and health conditions on the one hand, and the extent of urban planning activities on the other. Two sets of data were collected. The first consists of urban environmental variables, while the second consists of urban planning variables. The two sets are compared descriptively with respect to various contiguous parts of the city.

Findings from the study show that urban environmental health conditions and urban planning activities are closely related. The more intensive the planning activities the higher the level of environmental sanitation status in regard to various areas of the city.

Emerging from the study as a policy implication is the need to intensify efforts in urban planning as a key approach in ameliorating undesirable environmental health conditions of the cities.

Introduction

According to United Nations estimates, the proportion of world population that will live in urban areas will have increased to about 50 per cent by the year 2000, and cities with more than 10 million inhabitants will be common place (United Nations, 1985). This development will have the greatest impact in the developing countries, where the most rapid increases are occurring.

The poor state of living condition in most cities of the developing countries has been a subject of concern to physical planners. Despite the fact that a substantial share of the total population live and earn their living in the urban centres, adequate planning efforts are not made towards creating a conducive environment as well as improving the living condition of the urban populace. The generally intolerable urban environmental living conditions are overcrowding, lack of potable water supply, inadequate drains, absence and/or inadequate waste disposal facilities, air pollution, all of which are precipitating factors of various diseases.

Yet the relationship between urban planning and health dates back to the ancient Greeks and Romans who promoted the orderly arrangement of houses and streets as well as providing water as a means to prevent diseases and control them. More recently, in the United Kingdom, concern for the health of people who crowded into the major cities during the industrial revolution gave rise to housing regulations which evolved into health regulations, and eventually became the town and country planning laws (Egunjobi, 1991).

In Nigeria, modern town planning activities were triggered by bubonic plague which hit Lagos in 1924. Besides the immediate measures taken, the epidemic brought into being the Lagos Executive Development Board, which pioneered the development of new housing estates after demolishing some of the worst slums. However, some seven decades after this development, physical planning activities are still at the rudimentary stage, while urban environmental living conditions have stagnated or at best minimally improved in the country.

The objective of this paper is to highlight the association between urban environmental health conditions and physical planning activities, focusing on the city of Ibadan as an example.

Four neighbourhoods were selected on the basis of stratification for this study. The selected areas are Isale Foko, Mokola, Government Reservation Area (GRA), and Ojoo. The areas respectively correspond with the old core zone of the city, the newer zone, the exclusive zone and the periphery.

Two sets of data are presented:

The first consists of urban environmental variables which include 'population density', 'water supply' and 'toilet facilities'. The second set consists of urban planning variables and these include 'layout design', 'vehicular accessibility' and 'buildings subjected to approved plans'.

Environmental health variables

In Tables 6.1 to 6.3 are presented information relating to urban environmental health in the four selected study areas in Ibadan. Table 6.1, which highlights aspects of population density, shows that 86.9%, 36.9%, 24.6% and 17.1% of the houses sampled in GRA, transition zone, sub-urban zone and core area respectively meet the minimum occupancy ratio standard of 2 persons per room. The remaining proportions in the four areas have occupancy ratios of more than two persons per room which is an indication of a degree of over-crowding. The problem of human over-crowding therefore is more pronounced in the core area while it is least pronounced in the GRA.

From Table 6.2, the same pattern of better urban environmental health conditions in the GRA and the Transition Zone relative to the situation in the Sub-Urban and Core Zones is observed. If categories of respondents with 'piped water in house', 'piped water in community' and 'protected wells' are assumed as having safe water to drink, the highest proportion of 95.7% is found in the GRA. This is followed by respondents in the Transition Zone with 92.6%. A relatively lower proportion of 73.4% indicates safe water conditions in the Core Area, while the lowest proportion of 63.0% came from the Sub-Urban Area. It can be observed that the sample residents of the GRA also have the highest proportion of in-house piped water; while those in the core area appear more exposed to water from unsafe sources (i.e. unprotected wells and streams/brooks).

Table 6.1
Population densities in Ibadan

Room Occupancy	Core No.	%	Transitional No.	%	GRA No.	%	Sub-Urban No.	%
Average of 1 person/room	2	1.9	2	4.3	9	39.1	-	-
Average of 2 persons/room	16	15.2	15	32.6	11	47.8	14	24.6
Average of 3 persons/room	60	57.1	10	21.7	1	43.0	23	40.4
Average of 4 persons/room	27	25.07	14	30.4	-	-	18	31.6
Average of 5 persons/room	-	-	4	8.7	-	-	2	3.5
Average of 6 persons/room	-	-	1	2.2	1	4.3	-	-
No response	-	-	-	-	-	1.0	-	-
Total	105	100.0	46	100.0	23	100.0	57	100.0

Source: Field Survey, 1989.

Table 6.2

Sources of water supply in Ibadan

Sources of water supply	Core No.	%	Transitional No.	%	GRA No.	%	Sub-Urban No.	%
Piped water in house	13	12.4	27	58.7	18	78.3	20	35.1
Piped water in community	63	60.0	11	23.9	-	-	1	1.8
Protected wells	1	1.0	-	-	4	17.4	15	26.1
Unprotected wells	23	21.9	8	17.7	1	4.3	19	33.3
Stream/brook	5	4.8	-	-	-	-	1	1.8
No response	-	-	-	-	-	-	1	1.8

Source: Field Survey, 1989

Table 6.3

Types of toilet facility in Ibadan

Types of toilet	Core No.	%	Transitional No.	%	GRA No.	%	Sub-Urban No.	%
Water closet	10	9.5	30	62.5	23	100.0	20	35.1
Pit latrine	63	60.0	16	348	-	-	26	45.6
Bucket latrine	5	4.8	-	-	-	-	1	1.8
Open space/bush	5	4.8	-	-	-	-	7	12.3
No where in particular	22	21.0	-	-	-	-	3	5.3
Total	105	100.0	46	100.0	23	100.0	57	100.0

Source: Field Survey, 1989

The situation of human waste disposal is depicted in Table 6.3. Again, the disparity between the GRA and other sampled zones is clearly shown. Whereas every house that was sampled in the GRA had water closest toilets, the proportions with this facility vary from 9.5% in the core area to 65.2% in the Transition Zone. It is noteworthy that the bucket latrine system is still in use in some parts of the core zone (4.8%) and sub-urban zone (1.8%). However, the most undesirable situation is found in the Core and sub-urban zones where 21.0% and 5.3% respectively defecate in no particular places.

Physical planning variables

Tables 6.4 to 6.6 show the situation of town planning activities in the four zonal areas studied. The data presented in Table 6.4 show that all the houses sampled in the GRA were built within the framework of a layout design. This is to say that the whole of this area was subjected to proper town planning principles. On the other hand, only 3.8% and 29.8% were respectively found in the core and sub-urban areas as having been built within the framework of particular layout designs.

The level of planning activities is further illustrated in Table 6.5 where, again, the GRA houses are all accessible to vehicles. The transition zone also shows a relatively high degree of accessibility (73.9%) and the sub-urban zone 52.6%) with the core area exhibiting the lowest level of accessibility.

The picture that emerges in Table 6.6 is akin to what has been observed in the previous two tables. It shows further the intensity of physical planning activities in the various structural zones of the city. The GRA once again exhibits the highest degree of planning influence where 95.7% sought for and obtained planning approval for their residential buildings. This is followed by the transition zone with 82.6% of the building plans approved, and 54.4% in the Sub-Urban Zone. The Core Area is associated with the lowest proportion of 29.5%.

Discussion

A comparison of the two sets of data (i.e the data in Tables 6.1 - 6.3 and those in Tables 6.4 - 6.6) shows that the most deplorable environmental conditions are found in the core Area of the city. On the other hand, the GRA exhibits the highest level of environmental health status. At the same time, it is the core area where there is the lowest level of planning activities. That is to say the area evolved without being subjected to town planning principles and practice. This is in contrast to the GRA which is conceived within a planning framework and where development control is an on-going activity.

The GRA and the core area represent the two extreme situations which show that there is possibly a close association between planning variables and urban environmental health variables. The association which is yet to be subjected to statistical testing indicates that the more intensive the planning activities, the higher the level of environmental sanitation status with regard to various structural areas of the cities.

Table 6.4

Is your house within a designed layout?

Responses	Core		Transitional		GRA		Sub-Urban	
	No.	%	No.	%	No.	%	No.	%
Yes	4	3.8	-	-	23	100.0	17	29.8
No	100	95.2	17	37.0	-	-	39	68.4
No response	1	1.0	-	-	-	-	1	1.8
Total	105	100.0	46	100.0	23	100.0	57	100.0

Source: Field Survey, 1989

Tables 6.5

Is your house accessible to vehicular traffic?

Responses	Core		Transitional		GRA		Sub-Urban	
	No.	%	No.	%	No.	%	No.	%
Yes	28	26.7	34	73.9	23	100.0	30	52.6
No	77	73.3	12	26.1	-	-	26	45.6
No response	-	-	-	-	-	-	1	1.8
Total	105	100.0	46	100.0	23	100.0	57	100.0

Source: Field Survey, 1989

Table 6.6

Was an approval obtained in respect of this house?

Responses	Core		Transitional		GRA		Sub-Urban	
	No.	%	No.	%	No.	%	No.	%
Yes	31	29.5	38	82.6	22	95.7	31	54.4
No	72	67.6	8	17.4	1	4.3	25	43.9
No response	3	2.9	-	-	-	-	1	1.8
Total	105	100.0	46	100.0	23	100.0	57	100.0

Source: Field Survey, 1989

Although such an exercise (statistical test) is considered necessary, it is perhaps sufficient at this juncture to point to some relevant areas of the literature where the links between the variables have variously been linked to the conditions of health.

For example, living structures have been conceived as important artifacts in the urban environment. Mandelker and Montgomery (1973) believe that houses and health are inseparable. However, there is a dearth of research in this regard in the less developed countries (Tipple and Hellen, 1986, 1991). One of the most important housing infrastructure that is closely linked with health and disease are water supply and sanitation facilities. Water quality is essential to limit direct transmission of pathogens and epidemic (e.g. of cholera). At the same time, Stephen *et al*; (1985) contends that improvements in water supply and sanitation are unlikely to provide full and effective health protection in the absence of other socio-economic improvements.

One other aspect of the urban environmental condition that is closely related to ill-health is high population density. Calhou's (1965) experiment on animal colonies revealed that high densities might lead to pathological behaviour. From the experiment, he deduced that high population density promotes aggression, disrupts normal mating, nesting and material activities. He also linked spontaneous abortion, higher rates of illness and death to density. On human beings, it has been confirmed that home density and pathology are directly related (Sommer, 1966; Galle *et al;* 1972). Schmitt (1966) has also linked the problem of over-crowding with infant mortality and infectious disease incidences. Crowding brings about higher chances of interpersonal contacts thus enhancing chances of transmission of communicable diseases and triggering of mental illness Stephen *et al.*,(1985) while Odango (1978) has associated it with the spread of typhoid and tuberculosis. There is increasing evidence of the close relationship between TB and housing on recent reports on resurgence of TB in Zambia.

As pointed out in the introductory section, the close association between environmental health problems and planning activities is not new. In 1842; Edwin Chadwick produced a report on sanitary condition of the labouring population of Britain (cited in Macpherson, 1974). In the report, Chadwick asserted that diseases and poor life expectancy were associated with poor housing and other pathologies or environmental risk containers (ERC). These include over-crowding, poor sanitary services, poor drainage and poor water services. Where these are ameliorated, improvement in health and morale of the communities often follow. In the same line, Benevolo (1980) affirms that the Public Health Acts of Britain (1846) and that of France (1850), all of which aimed at improved housing, were effective enough to combat epidemic outbreak of cholera in these countries.

Conclusion

Emerging from this study as a policy implication is the need to intensify efforts in urban planning activities as a key approach in ameliorating undesirable health conditions in the cities. Urban planning as a field of study and as a profession possesses those technical attributes, methodological approaches and legislative measures which are capable of enhancing the physical, social and economic quality of the urban environment.

References

Benevolo, Leonardo (1980). *The Origin of Modern Town Planning.* The MIT Press. Mass. USA.

Calhoun, J.B. (1962). 'Population Density and Social Pathology'; *Scientific American*, Vol. 206, pp. 139-148.

Egunjobi, Layi (1991). 'Tackling Africa's Slums', in *World Health*, March-April; Geneva.

Galle, O., Gore, R. and Macpherson, J. (1972). 'Population Density and Pathology: What Relationships for Man?' *Journal of Health and Social Behaviour*, vol. 14, pp. 209-230.

Hellen, J.A., Tipple A.G. and Prince, M.A. (1991). Environmental risk assessment in a tropical city: an application of housing and household data from Kumasi, Ghana, in Hinz, E. (Editor) *Geomedizinische and biogeographische Aspekie der Krankheitsverbreilung und gesundheits verorging in Industrie-und Entwicklungslandern*. Frankfurt.

Macpherson, Ron (1974). 'Housing and Health: Some Basic Principles', in H. Murison and P. Lea (eds) *Housing in the Third World Countries: Perspectives on Policy and Practice*, Hong Kong: Macmillan Press Ltd., pp. 67-82.

Mandelker, D.R. and Montgomery, R. (1973). *Housing in America: Problems and Perspectives*. New York: Bobbs-Merril Company Inc.

Odango, John (1978). "Housing Deficits in Cities of the Third World: Fact or Fiction?" In Murison, H and P. Lea (eds.) *Housing in the Third World Countries: Perspectives on Policy and Practice*; Hong Kong: Macmillan Press Ltd.

Sommer, R. (1966). 'Man's Proximate Environment'; *Journal of Social Issues*, Vol. 22, pp. 59-70.

Stephens, B., Mason, J.P. and Isely, R. (1985). 'Health and Low Cost Housing', *World Health Forum*, 6: 59-62.

Tipple, A.G. and Hellen, J.A. (1986). *Priorities for Public Utilities and Housing Improvements in Kumasi, Ghana: An Empirical Assessment Based on Six Variables;* 'Seminar Papers' No. 44; Dept of Geography, University of Newcastle-Upon-Tyne.

7 Urban health hazards in Srinagar, India

Rais Akhtar

Summary

Health conditions in urban areas are the reflection of not only the availability of medical facilities but also the sanitation, transport network, levels of pollution, housing conditions, overcrowding as well as availability of recreational facilities. The paper is aimed at the assessment of residents' perception concerning health hazards which affects the health of the people in different areas. The levels of perception and its impact on people's behaviour varies over time and space. This variation is no doubt related to the socio-cultural and economic background, and the geography of the particular areas. Three localities in Srinagar urban area have been selected in order to study how the residents perceive the health hazards of their locality; identify the variation in their perception if any; and what particular health hazard most or least concerned the residuals. It is hoped that such studies based on local field studies may contribute significantly in urban health planning.

Introduction

Man's concern about his environment stems from the threat that environmental pollution poses to his comfort, health and existence (Meade, Florin and Gestler 1988). Increased awareness and concern are not limited to the problems of air and water pollution. Discussion of problems of the urban environment, of outdoor recreation, and of threatened animal species appeared with increasing frequency in newspapers and magazines and on radio and television. The discussion has extended to all the problems, present and anticipated that result from rapid growth of population, urbanization, industrialization, and affluence (Saarinen, 1976). In developed countries, like the United States, public opinion polls were conducted in order to measure people's attitudes towards environment. One such study carried out in the United States revealed that "the strongest single factor for predicting environmental concern would appear to be educational level.

The more highly educated express greater environmental concern. The less educated and those of lower socio-economic status have the highest proportion who are not very concerned. This lower level of concern among the less affluent may result from their focus on other more pressing problems they must deal with each day (Saarine, 1976). A number of papers have appeared concerning the geographical perspective of health and health care in urban area. The major emphasis in such studies has been placed on the spatial patterning of ill-health and mortality, physical and human environmental correlates and the organization of health care. However, there exists hardly any work on the understanding of people's perception of health hazards in urban area. Some geographical works which are partially related to the theme includes the work of A. Desai and P.P. Karan. A. Desai focuses her attention on the measurement of perception and its impact on human behaviour in different socio-economic communities in Ahmedabad, India. (Desai, 1981) P.P. Karan has made an attempt to measure the people's awareness in his study carried out in Calcutta, India (Karan, 1980, 1981). The author of this paper carried out a study in Lusaka, Zambia in 1984 with the objective of assessing the variation in perception of urban health hazards in two socio-economically different localities (Akhtar, 1988).

Objectives

The main objective of the present study conducted in Srinagar, India (Fig. 7.1) is to focus on the assessment of urban health hazards by people. From the viewpoint of neighbourhood planning, it is desirable to know the differential perception of communities living in socio-economically different residential areas. Their awareness about environmental problems and their willingness to participate in the development programmes can go a long way in improving the health conditions of people living in urban areas.

Methodology

Perception is individualistic and changeable. However, if residents identify themselves with a group and share common beliefs and values, there is a possibility of the emergence of a general pattern in perception and behaviour (Desai, 1981). Data have been collected through a questionnaire pertaining to the subjective images of residents and objective images of investigators with the environmental quality. The environmental quality of each selected (stratified random) household and its surrounding area is evaluated with a score on a five-point scale (i.e. very poor, poor, fair, good, very good) by residents and investigators. This assessment of environmental quality is based on pre-determined variables, including the general appearance and cleanliness of the area, crowding, air pollution, traffic density, housing conditions and presence of mosquitoes and flies. The study is based on 98 households selected from three socio-economically different areas

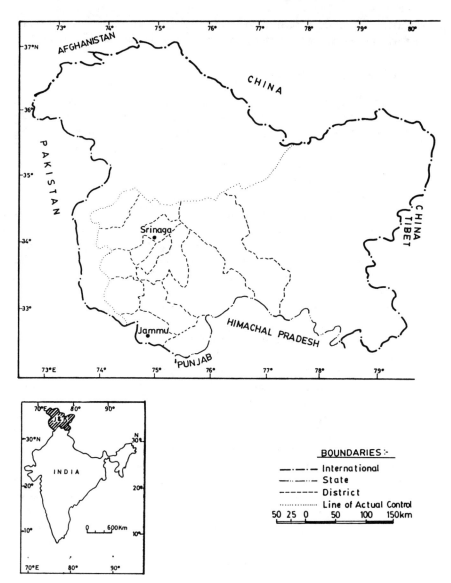

Figure 7.1   Jammu and Kashmir [Location map]

of Srinagar. An assessment of environmental health hazard has been made by computing response percentage on a five point scale for each variable. Besides this, the level of concern pertaining to the environmental quality has also been assessed on a five point

73

scale (deeply concerned, concerned, somewhat concerned, not concerned and no opinion). Response percentage to total for each of the eight indicators have been computed.

Urban ecology of the study area

The city of Srinagar (M.C.) covers an area of about 177.25 sq. km with a population of 570,195 giving a density of about 3,555 persons per sq.km. The land use pattern of the city shows that the built-up area includes 78.69 sq. km. (44.37 %) while the remaining non-built-up areas are covered by the lakes, rivers, nalas, marshy lands, orchards, agricultural lands and graveyards and so on (Fig. 7.2) Thus the built-up area remains very limited while the pressure of population on limited land grows year after year.

The main physiographic characteristics of the site and situation of Srinagar are such that the population is heavily concentrated along both the sides of the river Jhelum and in the adjoining areas. Because of the paucity of residential lands, the population of the city spills over in the low-lying areas, on the slopes of the ridges (Shankara Charya, the Itari Parvat and the Zansker range facing the Dal lake), as well as on the surface of the water bodies (The Dal Lake, the bank of the river Jhelum and the nalas). The residential houses situated in these areas are faced by a number of problems, e.g. drinking water, drainage, sewerage and so on. These problems become more acute during the winter months.

The water-borne diseases are thus more common among the *hanjis* who lives in houseboats and also among the dwellers of the slopping areas where potable water is not available.

The population which is heavily concentrated along the river Jhelum forms compact residential areas. These areas are called the "core areas" of the city. These areas which bear the characteristics of zig-zag roads, narrow lanes, by lanes, dilapidated houses, vertical structures, drainage and sewerage problems, inadequate public amenities and facilities - are some of the major problems which affect the health of the population.

The formation of the core areas is not new to Srinagar alone; it developed in almost all the cities of the medieval period. In the recent past, a large scale of exodus from the rural areas has further aggravated the situation over the already congested dwelling so much so that the core areas have become the plethora of urban problems: overcrowding slums, drainage, lack of civic amenities and facilities. Because of the problem of overcrowding, a number of families have started shifting to the outskirts of the city recently. Demographically the areas are over-populated by the fact that an area of 5 sq.km accounts for more than 50% of the total population of Srinagar. According to our estimate, there is a density of 44,000 per sq. kilometre in the core areas including, Rainawari locality, as compared to 1,910 in other parts of the city. This high density can be explained from a cultural perspective. There is a strong tradition of living together in a joint family, and children are greatly attached to their parents. There are rare exceptions where children live separately after their marriage. This has led to overcrowding in the families.

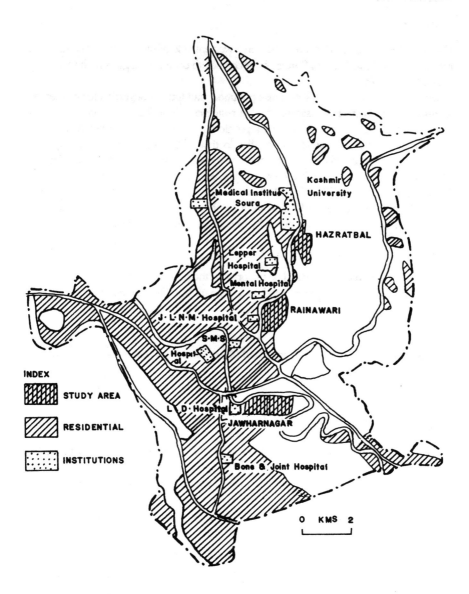

INDEX

▨ STUDY AREA

▧ RESIDENTIAL

▒ INSTITUTIONS

0 KMS 2

Figure 7.2   Srinagar city [Location of study area]

Analysis of data

Hazratbal:

Hazratbal locality is situated along the north-western side of the famous Dal Lake. The area is famous for its Muslim Shrine. An urban health centre and a girl's high school are located in the area.

The movement on the roadside, noise pollution, and traffic congestion have emerged as major health hazards as assessed by the residents (Table 7.1). Since no industry is located in this area, air-pollution is not a problem in Hazratbal. The assessment by the investigator is to some extent also similar to that of the residents. (Table 7.2). The investigator has assessed as 'poor' most of the health hazards as well as the availability of amenities in the locality. Table 7.3 reveals the level of concern pertaining to different health hazards. Nearly 67% of residents are 'deeply concerned' about cleanliness/sanitation. Generally people of the locality are either illiterate or less educated, hence they are unable to understand the danger posed by mosquitoes/flies as health hazard.

Rainawari

Rainawari is a high density area. The majority of the population is self-employed. One hospital as well as one high school and three primary schools are located in the area.

Table 7.1

Assessment by residents (Hazratbal) (% to total for a particular indicator)

	1	2	3	4	5	6	7	8	9	10	11	12
Very Poor	43.48	15.22	17.40	-	19.56	6.52	-	2.17	2.17	-	-	-
Poor	52.17	71.74	63.04	-	23.91	13.04	67.38	34.78	50.00	58.69	43.48	91.30
Fair	4.35	10.87	8.70	-	10.83	10.87	15.22	28.25	30.44	30.43	50.00	6.53
Good	-	2.17	4.35	-	26.10	39.13	15.22	26.10	10.87	8.71	4.35	2.17
Very Good	-	-	6.51	-	19.60	30.44	2.18	8.70	6.52	2.17	2.17	-

Table 7.2

Assessment by investigation (Hazratbal) (% to total for a particular indicator)

	1	2	3	4	5	6	7	8	9	10	11	12
Very Poor	47.83	23.91	15.22	-	6.52	-	2.17	2.17	2.17	-	-	-
Poor	52.17	65.22	58.69	6.52	21.74	43.48	56.54	54.34	60.87	63.04	78.26	73.91
Fair	-	6.53	4.35	2.17	15.22	15.22	30.43	32.61	30.43	30.43	15.21	17.39
Good	-	2.17	8.69	4.35	28.26	15.22	8.69	6.52	6.53	4.36	4.36	2.17
Very Good	-	2.17	13.05	86.96	28.26	26.08	2.17	4.36	-	2.17	2.17	6.53

Residents of the area assessed unhygienic conditions as a major health hazard, though at a lesser degree. With the exception of cleanliness-sanitation and traffic density, no other health hazard and the provision of amenities fall under the category of 'very poor' (Table 7.4). The investigator's assessment (Table 7.5) put cleanliness and sanitation under the 'poor' category and the allotted percentage as high as around 81. Cleanliness-sanitation and traffic density have been assessed as 'very poor' by the investigator. As regards the provision of amenities, both school and health facilities are fairly distributed in the locality. This is similar to the assessment made by the residents (Table 7.6). About residents' concern regarding various health hazards, nearly 81% are deeply concerned about the insanitary condition in the area. About 76 and 79% are also concerned about the poor housing condition as well as mosquitoes/flies in the area.

Table 7.3

To what extent are residents concerned about health hazards (Hazratbal) (% to total for a particular hazard)

	1	2	3	4	5	6	7	8
Deeply concerned	67.40	32.61	28.26	32.61	26.29	43.48	17.39	8.69
Concerned	23.91	28.26	39.15	19.56	19.39	32.61	39.13	32.62
Somewhat concerned	6.52	-	-	-	-	-	-	2.17
Not concerned	21.74	10.87	26.09	45.63	-	2.17	-	
No opinion	2.17	17.39	21.72	21.74	8.69	23.91	41.31	56.52

Table 7.4

Assessment by residents (Rainawari) (% to total for a particular indicator)

	1	2	3	4	5	6	7	8	9	10	11	12
Very Poor	21.42	-	2.38	-	-	-	-	-	-	-	-	-
Poor	52.00	52.38	47.62	-	35.72	23.81	33.33	28.57	28.57	28.57	28.57	28.57
Fair	7.14	35.72	40.48	-	30.95	23.81	40.48	57.15	57.15	52.42	57.15	52.42
Good	21.44	11.90	9.52	-	30.95	47.62	26.19	14.28	14.28	19.01	14.28	19.01
Very Good	-	-	-	-	2.38	4.76	-	-	-	-	-	-,

Jawahar Nagar

Jawahar Nagar is an upper middle class residential area. The majority of the population is highly educated and work for the government or private institutions. According to the assessment by residents (Table 7.7) cleanliness - sanitation is not a problem in the area. However, the residents consider noise and air pollution as hazards in the area. This is because of the fact that most people own their cars, as well as impact of air pollution.

Amenities such as transport, health and school are sufficiently available in the area. The roads are quite wide and thus no problem regarding the movement on the roadside. The investigator has not assessed any hazard and the provision of amenities under 'very poor' category (Table 7.8). Similar to the assessment made by residents, the investigator has also assessed hazard related to mosquito/flies as 'poor'. The assessment made by investigator shows that water pollution is a problem and categorised it as 'poor'. This is probably the impact of the pollutants from the industries. Amenities such as transport,

Table 7.5

Assessment by investigator (Srinagar Rainawari) (% to total for a particular indicator)

	1	2	3	4	5	6	7	8	9	10	11	12
Very poor	9.52	-	-	-	2.38	-	-	-	-	-	-	-
Poor	80.96	28.57	30.96	-	19.05	19.05	21.43	23.81	28.57	23.81	23.81	23.81
Fair	4.76	47.62	50.00	-	38.09	28.57	47.62	54.76	54.76	57.14	57.14	57.14
Good	2.38	19.05	14.28	-	33.34	52.38	28.57	21.43	16.67	19.05	19.05	19.05
Very good	2.38	4.76	4.76	-	7.14	-	2.38	-	-	-	-,-	

Table 7.6

To what extent are residents concerned about health hazards (Rainawari) (% to total for a particular hazard)

	1	2	3	4	5	6	7	8
Deeply concerned	80.96	33.34	54.76	-	-	38.09	4.76	2.38
Concerned	16.66	54.76	38.10, -	-	42.86	76.19	78.57	
Somewhat concerned	2.38	4.76	-	-	-	7.14	2.38	-
Not concerned	-	7.14	7.14	-	-	2.39	-	-
No opinion	-	-	-	-	-	9.52	16.67	19.05

Table 7.7

Assessment by residents (Jawahar Nagar) (% to total for a particular indicator)

	1	2	3	4	5	6	7	8
Very Poor	-	10	10	60	50	50	-	20
Poor	-	70	70	30	40	50	-	80
Fair	60	20	20	10	10	-	10	-
Good	38	-	-	-	-	-	70	-
Very Good	10	-	-	-	-	-	20	-

Table 7.8

Assessment by investigator (Jawahar Nagar)(% to total for a particular indicator)

	1	2	3	4	5	6	7	8
Very poor	-	-	-	-	30	-	-	-
Poor	-	70	60	80	40	90	-	80
Fair	40	30	40	20	30	10	30	20
60								
Good	50	-	-	-	-	-	50	-
Very good	10	-	-	-	-	-	20	-

health as well as movement on the roadside have been assessed as 'fair' by the investigator. Nearly 70% of residents are "deeply concerned" about the cleanliness-sanitation, while only 30% are 'somewhat concerned' about it (Table 7.9). Contrary to this only about 20% each are concerned with the problems related to traffic density and air pollution. About 70 and 60% are 'somewhat concerned' regarding the housing condition and mosquitoes/flies respectively.

Conclusion

The study was aimed at determining the seriousness of urban health hazards as perceived by the residents. The study reveals that range of individual perception of environmental quality varies to some extent in different areas. However, there are no significant variations between the assessment by the residents and the investigator. Also evident is the fact that residents assessed their environment not only as individuals but as an entire community. The study also highlights the fact that the variations in the assessment of health hazards

Table 7.9
To what extent residents are concerned about health hazards (Jawahar Nagar)
(% to total for a particular hazard)

	1	2	3	4	5	6	7	8
Deeply concerned	70	-	20	20	-	-	30	-
Concerned	-	-	-	-	-	-	-	-
Somewhat concerned	30	50	30	50	-	20	70	60
Not very concerned	-	20	50	30	-	40	-	40
No opinion	-	30	-	-	100	40	-	-

is the relation of the socio-economic structure of the population concerned. The economically and educationally well off assessed noise and air pollution as health hazards while they are quite 'deeply concerned' with cleanliness-sanitation. Contrary to this, residents in other medium and high-density areas assessed unhygienic environment and traffic density as a health hazard.

Besides this, the description of data concerning the people's perception, their housing conditions and their locality, the availability of amenities in the area may be useful in the socio-economic health planning of the area concerned. It must be added that the core area development programme being initiated in Srinagar is aimed at the development of parks, removal of slums, widening of roads, repair and replacement of old bridges. These measures if implemented may considerably reduce the unhygienic conditions in urban Srinagar.

Acknowledgement

I am grateful to my post-graduate students and research scholars who assisted me in obtaining data. Also I am thankful to Dr. M. Siddiq for his comments on aspects of urban ecology of Srinagar.

References

Akhtar, R. (1988). Perception of Urban Health Hazards: Examples from Lusaka, Zambia, *International Journal of Environmental Studies*, 31. 2-3, pp. 167-172

Desai, A. (1981). 'Differential Perception of Residents to Environmental Quality of an Urban Area: The Case of Ahmedabad', *Geographical Review of India*, 43, 2, pp. 156-165, pp. 198-199

Karan, P.P. (1980-82). Public Awareness of Environmental problems in Calcutta Metropolitan Area', *National Geographical Journal of India*, 26-28, pp. 29-34.

Meade, M., Florin, J. and Gestler, W. (1988). *Medical Geography*, New York, The Guilford Press p. 167.

Saarinen, T.F., (1976). *Environmental Planning: Perception and Behaviour* , Atlanta, Houghton Mifflin Company, p. 198.

8 Environmental health in low income settlements: A preliminary survey of health issues in the city of Colombo, Sri Lanka

Y. A. D. S. Wanasinghe

Summary

The quality of a dwelling and its immediate environment as well as the availability of amenities affect the physical and mental health of human beings. Although the inadequacy of facilities and environmental pollution in most parts of Colombo have an impact on the health of its residents it is the people living in low income settlements who are more exposed to health hazards.

In 1978, approximately 50% of the population in Colombo lived in slums and squatter settlements or shanties. Although attempts such as upgrading and sites and services projects have succeeded in improving the quality of some of the low income settlements, nearly 9000 unauthorized shanty units still remain to be developed.

These shanties are sited on or near already polluted areas in the city such as garbage dumps, marshes and canal reservations. The majority of shanty units are small huts with a high occupancy rate. Poor ventilation and the use of biomass fuels for cooking cause severe indoor pollution and due to overcrowding, communicable diseases are transmitted quickly. Water supply and toilet facilities are not adequate to ensure proper personal and domestic hygiene and there are no facilities for the disposal of solid waste.

An in-depth survey in 1991 of shanties in North Colombo revealed that there are several large concentrations in the area. At Aluthmawatha, 504 shanty units with a population of 3300 were severed by 5 stand pipes and 12 public toilets. Hence shanty dwellers had constructed 74 temporary latrines in close proximity to 12 unauthorized dug wells. At Mahawatta, there were 3 main concentration with a total of 461 units. They were provided with 7 stand pipes and 4 public toilets. Three temporary latrines were constructed by the squatters for adults while children generally defecated on the ground outside the huts or along the canal. Improper location of latrines, in relation to wells, defecation on the ground, frequent flooding and waterlogged conditions in these areas have resulted in the biological contamination of food, water and soil. As a result, in addition to the respiratory diseases, gasteritis and infective diseases prevalent in the area there was an outbreak of cholera in North Colombo in 1991.

Introduction

The quality of dwellings, characteristics of their indoor and outdoor environment and the availability of amenities can have a strong impact on the physical and mental health of human beings. The urban poor, residing in slums and squatter settlements that are located in polluted environments without any adequate or safe water supply and means for sanitary disposal of solid waste and excreta, are more vulnerable to health than other residents in urban areas.

The city of Colombo had an estimated population of 625,000 in 1991. Although growth rates of population in Colombo have declined in recent years, the number who live in slums and squatter settlements (known as shanties in Sri Lanka) has increased. In 1978, they constituted 50% of the city population. By the end of 1987, however, slum upgrading and sites and services projects have reduced the number of substandard dwellings. As indicated in Table 8.1 only 8846 of shanty units housing a total population of 45,840 remained to be improved by 1987. As much as 54% of these shanties are located in Northern and Central Colombo. (Fig.8.1)

Health situation of shanty dwellers

Morbidity and mortality figures available for environmentally-related diseases in the Government hospitals within the city, (used primarily by the low income population) reveal that there is a high incidence of intestinal infections such as shigellosis, amoebiosis, ancylostomiasis helminthiasis etc. among the patients. Respiratory diseases, Japanese encephalitis, viral hepatitis, dengue haemorrhagic fever (DHF), filariasis and cholera are the other diseases for which people had come for treatment. Among the shanty dwellers, the most common ailments are respiratory diseases and bowel disorders (Table 8.2). Colombo is located within the endemic belt for urban filariasis and it has a comparatively high micro-filarial rate of 1.7% but the wards with a large concentration of shanties had a higher rate of 3%. The presence of dengue vectors - *Aedes aegypti* and *A. albopictus* around shanty communities can also be attributed to the poor environmental conditions in low income communities. Dengue was first detected in the 1960s but had remained dormant for a long time. Today a more virulent strain has been detected in Colombo. The danger lies in the fact that the vector Aedes aegypti breeds in fresh water collected in coconut shells, flower vases, polythene bags and discarded household utensils in home gardens and garbage dumps. Their eggs can survive in an area with very little moisture even for 6 months.

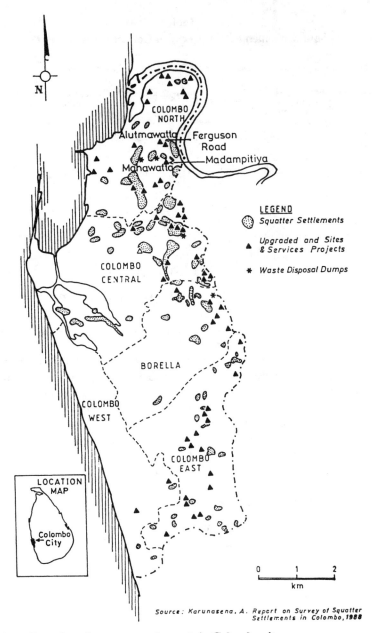

Figure 8.1   Location of squatter settlements in Colombo city

Table 8.1
Squatter settlements in the city of Colombo, December 1987

Electorate	No. of units improved by December 1987					No. of units not improved			
	No. of projects	No. of units	No. of families	Popula-tion	%	No. of units	No. of families	Popula-tion	%
Colombo North	18	3746	4,447	22949	35.6	1859	2164	9366	20.4
Colombo Central	13	2283	2,642	14794	23.0	2924	3615	15773	34.4
Colombo West	03	428	512	2684	4.1	1902	2321	9962	21.7
Colombo East	13	2315	2,555	13287	20.7	1722	2001	8557	18.7
Borella	08	1858	2051	10663	16.5	439	491	2182	4.8
Total	55	10625	12207	64337	100.0	8846	10592	45840	100.0

Source: A. 'Karunasena, Report on the Survey of Squatter Settlements in the Colombo City, 1988. p.24.

Very few cholera cases were reported after 1976 but in 1991 there was a cholera epidemic which originated in the shanty community at Mahawatta in Colombo North. The first patient belonged to a squatter family that lived along the railway reservation where basic amenities such as water and latrines were not available. Cholera is transmitted by the faecal-oral route from person to person. A few days later, cholera spread to the adjoining shanty communities at Madampitiya road and Ferguson road and thence to other shanties in Colombo (Fig. 8.1). As indicated in Table 8.3, the epidemic which reached its peak in August, 1991 was confined to Colombo and its immediate suburbs.

Outdoor environment of shanties and its relationship to health

The city of Colombo is served with pipe-borne water and by a sewerage system which is at present overloaded. Until recently 68,000 - 90,000 cubic meters of raw sewage and industrial waste per day was discharged into the sea and to the estuary of river Kelani which forms the northern boundary of the City of Colombo. A daily organic load of 10,000 - 24000 kg BOD 5/d therefore entered the river from this source (NARESA, 1991). Sewage and industrial effluents are also discharged into the city's canal network, lagoons and small lakes such as the Beira, Study of water quality (NARESA, 1991) of outfalls from which the Beira lake receives city waste revealed that COD levels vary between 29 and 816 mg/1 and SS in the range of 39 - 33 mg/1.

The city of Colombo has a high air pollution level. Results of air quality monitoring revealed that sulphation rates ranged between 0.04 and 0.45 milligrams per 100 square centimetres, (NARESA, 1991) especially in the major commercial areas. Sulphation rate is measured by the concentration of sulphur compounds such as sulphur dioxide, sulphur trioxide and hydrogen sulphide in the atmosphere. High levels

Table 8.2

Morbidity in selected squatter settlements during August 1982

Name of ailment	Age group					All ages
	Under 1 year	1-5 years	6-14 years	15-60 years	Over 60 years	
1. Respiratory diseases	68.75	59.84	66.67	58.17	18.75	60.52
2. Gastroenteritis	9.38	25.98	23.19	15.69	6.25	19.96
3. Common infective diseases	9.38	6.30	5.80	0.65	-	4.29
4. Heart diseases	3.12	0.79	-	6.54	25.00	3.43
5. Accidents and poisonings	-	0.79	0.72	3.27	12.50	1.93
6. Skin diseases	6.25	6.30	-	3.92	-	3.43
7. Cancer	-	-	-	1.81	-	0.43
8. Rheumatic diseases	3.12			4.58	-	1.72
9. All other diseases	-	-	3.62	5.87	37.50	4.29
Percentage for all diseases by specific age groups	100.00	100.00	100.00	100.00	100.00	100.00
Percentage of those reporting ill by age groups	6.88	27.25	29.61	32.83	3.43	100.00

Source: Marga Institute, Colombo City Information Document, 1982 (in the Appendix)

lead to the aggravation of respiratory diseases and eye infections and impairment of visibility. Dustfall is measured by the total settleable dust in the atmosphere. At major traffic intersections in Colombo, dustfall is over 300 milligrams per square meter per day and around industrial areas a rate of over 1400 mg/sq. meter/day has been recorded. The presence of lead in urban dust too has an adverse effect on human health.

Shanty dwellers are more at risk than other city residents and commuters since their huts are located in the most polluted areas in the city. Shanties are sited along canal, river, road and railway reservations, on marshy and water logged areas in the city's periphery and on or near garbage dumps. As illustrated in Fig. 8.2, 76 of the shanty communities (clusters) are located along the city's canal net work. They have been described as "open sewers", since domestic and solid waste from shanties

Table 8.3
Distribution of cholera cases June and August 1991

Location	No. of Cases	
	June	August
I. Colombo		
Shanty communities in		
(a) Aluthmawatha		03
(b) Bloemendhal		04
(c) Ferguson Road		,
Magalagam Road	28	10
Madampitiya Road		,
(d) Other Shanty Communities	00	34
II. Suburbs of Colombo	2	17
III. Other parts of Sri Lanka	60	68
Total for Sri Lanka	30	68

Source: Bulletin of Communicable Diseases, Weekly Epidemiological Report Dept. of Health, 1991 August.

are dumped into canals. Of the total waster load discharged into the canals, 50-60% comprise sewage. The large number of factories situated along the canals also discharge as much as 3900 Kg BOD 5/day. Canal water is stagnant or slow moving and water in some canals have been described as "highly turbid with an appreciable amount of sediments and flocculent matter in suspension". People living on low-lying marshy areas that are liable to frequent flooding also face health risks.

Other shanties are located on former garbage dumps or near existing ones. There are over 200 secondary collecting points in the city and several large refuse disposal points in the periphery. Refuse dumps have a short life span and new locations have to be selected every 3 or 6 months. They are not covered daily with soil and refuse is burnt at least once a week. The health conditions of shanty dwellers in the immediate vicinity of these dumps are affected as a result of:

    –   air pollution from smoke, ash, dust and air borne litter;

    –   contamination of surface and ground water through direct placement of wastes in marshes and through run-off leaking to streams; the movement of leachate through rock and soil to shallows ground water aquifers;

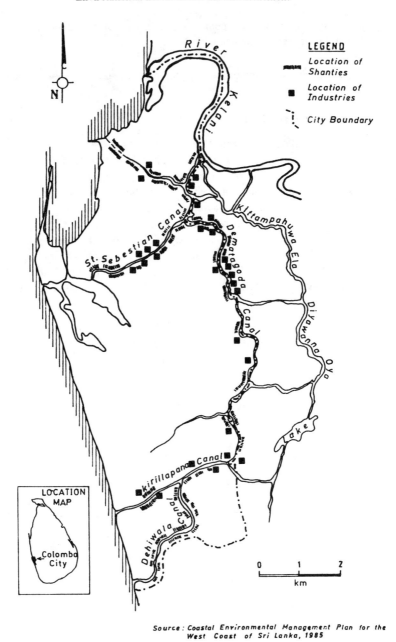

Source: Coastal Environmental Management Plan for the
West Coast of Sri Lanka, 1985

Figure 8.2   Location of shanties and factories along canals in Colombo city

- periodic flooding when contaminated water from the dumps spread to the neighbouring house sites.

-

- garbage dumps provide breeding places for disease carrying rodents, mosquitoes and flies.

Indoor environment of shanties

Shanties are small flimsy makeshift structures with temporary walls and roofs and dirt floors that harbour disease vectors. As depicted in Table 8.4, 86% of the shanties have a floor area below 300 square feet. Eighty percent of the shanty communities in North Colombo, however, are smaller units with a floor area below 200 square feet. The majority of huts are one roomed structures without proper windows. Light and ventilation is received through the doors or other openings in the walls that are protected by wire mesh. Sometimes gaps between the roof and the top of the walls or between planks that form the walls provide ventilation. Some shanties have a small kitchen separated from the living room. As reflected in Table 8.5, 93% of the shanty households in the sample used firewood for cooking and 5% used kerosene oil. The use of biomass fuels cause severe indoor pollution.

Table 8.4
Floor area of shanties in Colombo, 1987

Floor area per unit (sq.ft.)	No. of units						
	Colombo East	Colombo West	Borella	Colombo Central	Colombo North	Total no of units	%
Below 100	320	93	414	942	736	2,505	28.318
101-200	638	209	666	1165	713	3.391	38.334
201-300	355	80	479	556	304	1,774	20.054
Above 300	409	57	343	261	106	1,176	13.294
Total	1722	439	1902	2924	1859	8,846	100.00

Source: Karunasena, A., Report on the survey of squatter settlements in Colombo City, Colombo, 1988. p. 58

Various forms of respiratory diseases have been caused by air pollutants in these ill-ventilated shanties. The situation is exacerbated by poverty, malnutrition and over-crowding since as much as 45% of the shanties have more than 6 occupants living in a small area (Table 8.6). In North Colombo were there was a recent outbreak of cholera, the average occupancy rate exceeded 5 persons per unit (Karunasena, 1988) (Table 8.7). As pointed out in the WHO Report on Housing, "overcrowding particularly in conjunction with impoverished lifestyles and inadequate facilities has been implicated in transmission of tuberculosis, phenumonias, bronchitis and gastrointestinal infections, Airborne infections are encouraged when people sleep close together in poorly ventilated rooms" (WHO, 1987).

Table 8.5
Quality of dwellings of squatter settlements, Colombo, 1982

Housing units classified	Number	Percentage
i. *Fuel used for cooking*		
(a) firewood	629	93
(b) kerosene	34	5
(c) other	13	2
ii. *Water supply*		
(d) Private pipe	14	2
(e) Community pipe	640	93
(f) private well	5	1
(g) public well	24	4
iii. *Toilet facilities*		
(h) private latrine	12	2
(i) community latrine	407	63
(j) public latrine	124	19
(k) open space	104	16

Source: Marga Institute Inter - City Workshop on primary Health care in urban areas. Colombo City Information Document, 1982. pp.20 and 23

Access to facilities

The city of Colombo is served with pipe-borne water but the majority of shanty dwellers do not have easy access to a safe water supply. An adequate supply of safe potable water is essential to prevent the spread of gastro-intestinal diseases and to ensure personal and domestic hygiene. Over 90% of the shanty dwellers depend on roadside taps but each tap has to be shared among 100 families (500-600 people) and water has to be collected in buckets land pots from taps located one quarter of a mile away from the shanties which means that it is difficult to ensure good hygiene practices.

Table 8.6
Occupancy rate of shanties in Colombo, 1987.

Occupants per Unit	Electorate					Total no of units	Per cent
	Colombo East	Colombo West	Borella	Colombo Central	Colombo North		
1 - 5	68.41	68.34	64.72	60.74	65.95	5711	64.56
6 - 10	28.75	27.56	31.13	34.23	32.17	2807	31.73
11 - 15	2.26	3.87	3.84	4.62	1.83	298	3.37
Above 15	0.58	0.23	0.31	0.41	0.05	30	0.34
Total	100.00	100.00	100.00	100.00	100.00	8846	100.00

Source: Karunasena, A., Report on the survey of squatter settlements in the Colombo City, Colombo, 1988, p. 59.

Table 8.7
Occupancy rate in shanties in Colombo north, 1987

Name of ward where shanties are located	No. of units	No. of families	Total population	Persons per unit
Mattakkuliya	73	89	368	5.04
Modara	95	110	538	5.06
Mahawatta	459	518	2209	4.81
Aluthmawata	248	255	1077	4.34
Lunupokuna	99	129	561	5.06
Blomendhal	782	933	3995	5.10
Kotahena East	26	34	145	5.57
Kodtahena West	77	96	473	6.14
Total	1859	2164	9366	-

Source: Karunasena, A., Report on the survey of squatter settlements in the Colombo City, Colombo, 1988 p. 64.

Due to the absence of a sufficient number of taps, some squatters have dug wells to draw underground water. In highly congested areas in Colombo such as the Henamulla camp at Totalanga, pollution values in ground water have exceeded permissible levels land ranged from 24.0 to 53.2 mg/1 BOD6. Another study conducted in shanty areas at

Totalanga, Mattakkuliya and Kirulapone revealed that shallow wells in the area were grossly contaminated by faecal and organic matter. Further, high levels of nitrate which exceeded permissible levels of potable water were observed in deep wells. (Athukorale, 1985)

A field survey conducted in 1991 in selected shanty areas of Colombo North (Fig. 8.3) revealed that 5 taps had to be shared by 3300 people in the Aluthmawatha shanty community (Table 8.8) so that 12 wells had been constructed by the squatters to ensure a regular supply of water. Due to lack of space within the shanty community, these wells are sometimes dug within a 5 foot radius of the makeshift latrines. At Bloemendhal, 500 persons had to share 3 taps while 1120 people living in shanties along Ferguson road, Nagalagam road and Madampitiya road had to depend on 4 taps and one standpipe.

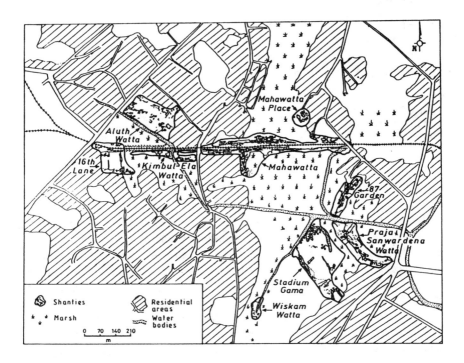

Figure 8.3   Squatter settlements in north Colombo

Table 8.8

Availability of amenities in selected shanty communities in Colombo north

Amenities and other characteristics	Aluth-mawatha	Bloemen dhal	Mahawatta Ferguson rd. Nagalagam rd. Madampitiya rd.	School garden	Praja Sanwarda nawatta
Housing units	504	88	383	59	19
Families	573	110	436	64	25
Population	3316	500	119	535	163
No. of taps	5	3	5	2	-
No. of unauthorized wells	12	-	-	-	-
No. of public latrines	12	6	4	-	-
No. of unauthorized make shift latrines	74	-	3	-	-

Source: Field Survey, 1991

The lack of a hygienic and acceptable method of excreta disposal also affects the health of shanty dwellers. As shown in Table 8.7, since 12 public latrines are not adequate to serve 330 in Aluthmawatha, the squatters had constructed 74 makeshift latrines. In other squatter communities children usually defecate outside the huts or along the canals. Due to the construction of latrines close to wells and to defecation on the ground, human faeces have become the main source of contamination of water and soil and the principal vehicle for the transmission and spread of a wide range of communicable diseases in shanty areas. During the rainy season, the insanitary conditions expose the shanty dwellers to helminthic and protozoal parasites. Contaminated water from the settlement sites in marshy areas usually flow to the nearby leafy vegetable plots ("keera" farms). Since shanty dwellers do not have facilities for the adequate and safe disposal of solid waste, garbage is either collected near the shanties and burnt regularly or thrown to the nearby canals, thus creating an environment suitable for the breeding of vectors, flies and rodents.

"Upgraded" squatter settlements and health

Through slum and shanty upgrading and sites and services projects, the Government, with assistance from UNICEF and NGOs, has attempted to improve the health situation of the urban poor. Today, there is a change in the perception of housing in Sri Lanka. There is an integrated programme and in the new concept, housing includes not only shelter but health, sanitation other amenities and services.

One of the important components of the UNICEF-assisted Environmental Health Community Development Project is the Health Education Programm (HEP) in the upgraded settlements. This programme is being implemented by Health Wardens and is aimed at increasing the health consciousness of the low income communities, creating positive attitudes towards health and sanitation; encouraging the communities to adopt improved health and hygiene practices and disseminating knowledge on health and sanitation. The evaluation of the phase 1 of the UNICEF project revealed that there has been a considerable improvement in preventive health care practices in areas where community participation through Community Development Councils as well as Volunteer Health Wardens was active. (Tilakaratna, et al; 1986)

Conclusion

This paper has attempted to show how inadequate housing and lack of basic amenities in urban low income settlements have an adverse impact on health. A certain measure of success has been achieved through slum and shanty upgrading and sites and services projects, where the improvement of the shelter, basic services and the physical environment has been complemented by the provision of health and nutrition education, child care facilities and by active community participation. A concerted effort has to be made, however, to upgrade the remaining squatter settlements in Colombo as well as others in the rapidly expanding suburbs in order to improve the health of the urban poor.

References

Athukorale, W.A.C. (1985). *Physio-Chemical and Microbiological Analysis of untreated Domestic Water supplies in and around Colombo* Reported at National Workshop on Environmental Health Research at Country Level Digana, Sri Lanka, 9 - 14 December 1985.

Fernando, R.V. Paulraj, P.J. and de Silva, M.A., (1985). *An Investigation of Faecal Pollution in water used for domestic purposes in 2 highly congested areas in and around the Municipal limits of Colombo*. Reported at the National Workshop on Environmental Health Research at country level, Digana, Sri Lanka, 9-14 December, 1985.

Karunasena, A. (1988). *Report on the Survey of Squatter settlements in Colombo*, Colombo.

National Building Research Organization, (1989): Quoted in NARESA, 1991, p. 90.

Natural Resources, Energy and Science Authority of Sri Lanka (NARESA), *Natural Resources of Sri Lanka*, Colombo, 1991, p. 164.

Tilakaratna, S., Hettige S., Karunaratne, W., (1986). "Environmental Health and Community Development Project. A case study in the slums and shanties of Colombo." Shabbir, Cheema (ed.) in *Reaching the Urban Poor* Westview Press Inc., Boulder, pp. 105-123.

WHO, *Housing - The Implications for Health*, Report of a WHO consultation, Geneva, 9-15 June, 1987.

9 Housing and health characteristics: An epidemological study of a tropical city

Tunde Agbola and O. A. Akinbamijo

Summary

Housing provision is subject to the laws of supply and demand, while quality and quantity consumed is a function of the consumers' effective demand. Given the socio-economic imbalances as regards infrastructural provisions, varying levels of disposable income and the relative immobility of housing, the housing market in Nigeria is typified by varying housing characteristics. These characteristics affect the types and incidences of various diseases in urban areas.

Many research works on urban living conditions confirm the existence of palpable relationships between housing and health. This paper examines the roles of tenement characteristics of the health of urban dwellers in a tropical city, Abeokuta.

Epidemiological analyses of randomly selected residential areas was done using percentiles and the analysis of variance (ANOVA) technique. The study indicates a significant relationship between tenement status and health potentialities of dwellers. Remedial measures recommended include enhanced maintenance culture.

Introduction

In most Nigerian cities, and for an increasing proportion of urban dwellers, the living conditions and the urban environment are rapidly deteriorating. Onibokun (1986) asserted that housing difficulties, especially for the low income groups have been complicated by conditions peculiar to developing countries with rapid growth, inflated real estate values, influx of poor immigrants and lack of planning, among other characteristics. This problem exists for both the urban and rural dwellers.

Abeokuta, the study area, is the political headquarters of Ogun state of Nigeria. The city has diversified natural features, prominent among which is the Olumo Rock. The prominence of this feature is reflected in the town's name which literally translates, "under the rock." Abeokuta is a conglomeration of villages, with Ake as the chief village (Johnson, 1897). It experiences tropical weather conditions with an elevation of 157 metres above sea level, and residual outcrops dotting the landscape.

The climate of the city is characterized by high rainfall, high temperature and high relative humidity. These conditions readily favour the proliferation of vectors and pathogens, causing various health problems.

The concept of health and housing

The improvement of the quality of life as one of the major objectives of urban development programmes identifies health status as a principal consideration in the planning and design of a house (Stephens *et al.*, 1985) and the housing programme itself. Stephens *et al.* also reveal varying strengths of association between housing features and certain health conditions. He affirmed the need to amplify health benefits of housing with a view to achieving maximum health effects from the units. Edwin Chadwick's '*Report on Sanitary conditions of the labouring population of Britain*' (1842, cited in Macpherson, 1979), ascertained the link between diseases and poor life expectancy as well as poor housing and other environmental risk containers.

With the foregoing, it is the goal of this paper to present its own understanding of health and housing. Kleevens (1983) asserted that the house forms part of the total environment where the greatest degree of family life is spent. Mahler (1981, D. General, WHO) argued later that "... it is there, where people live and work that health is made or broken. If health does not start with the individual, the home, ... we shall never get to the goal of Health for All" he added. These reveal the link between housing and health.

Mahler presented health as a state of personal well-being. It is a state that enables one to lead a socially and economically productive life. Macpherson (1979) saw health as that state involving a complete lack of morbidity - an opportunity to lead a fruitful existence peaceably. Akinbamijo (1988) presented health, however, as a dynamic state, attained in concert with environmental, social and economic forces. This paper therefore sees health as a concept, heterogeneous and holistic in nature. These properties allow health to be subjected to multisectoral analysis hence this paper probes the contribution of housing to health. Relevant literature also affirm that action taken outside the health sector can have health effects greater than those obtained within it, Mahler (1981); Macpherson (1979); Stephens *et al.*, (1985); Tipple and Hellen (1986, 1991) among others. Thus Akinbamijo (1988) believes that latent health enhancement resources exist in the housing sector. These, when exploited in the correct blend and harmony, lead to better health attainment.

Housing on the other hand, is viewed as a bundle of services that transcends mere shelter provision (Coleman Woobury, cited in Mandelker and Montgomery 1973). Wakely (1986) sees it as a range of goods and services that make up the domestic environment of a community of which shelter, is but a part. It is a process by which individuals and communities develop their environment and are influenced by it. Housing equates with developmental artefacts whose patterns determine the environmental quality of the town. These affect urban liveability and the reliability of the environment as a palpable predictor of urban liability to sicknesses and diseases. The virulent diseases such as tuberculosis had been on the decline even before the advent of medical therapy confirm the reliability on adequate environmental management as curative strategies. This is the basis of the maxim that urban renewal brings improvement on quality of life.

Decent housing is a basic need of Man. Housing needs and problems, however, permit the use of various structures and tenancy status. These are manifested in overcrowding, inadequate urban social amenities, unsatisfactory and unwholesome environmental conditions and urban squalor (Onibokun 1986). The cost implications of housing provision determine the operations and characteristics of the various housing submarkets on the urban-scapes.

Health and housing: a review of the literature

Many studies have been carried out on the relationships between health and housing. Fox (1972) cited in Tipple and Hellen (1986) ascertained that health and diseases are likely to be patterned according to the characteristics of housing zones of a district. He concluded that a knowledge of the environment could be used in effecting therapeutic strategies. Environmental risk containers when ameliorated, induce improvement in health. This lends credence to Dunlop's (1980) argument that bad housing have direct negative impact on the individuals' health. Benevolo (1980) affirmed the efficacy of Public Health Acts of Britain (in 1846) and France (in 1850) on the outbreak of cholera in the respective countries.

The effect of urban living on psychology of man has also been well studied. The effects of urbanization and psychological stress generated due to overcrowded, yet compartmentalized urban existence has been confirmed Agbola (1989); Galle et al. (1972); Wirth (1938). Schizoid mentality and segmental culture of the urbanite are credited to urban existence while neurotic any psychotic disorders, examined in different residential districts by Tsung - Yi - Lin (1959) reveal strong correlations between types of mental disorder and social/housing class.

Rheumatic heart disease, meningitis and some communicable diseases have greater chances of success due to ease of transmission in crowded housing (Stephens et al., (1985); Odongo (1978). Adequate land use planning and ordinances are capable of controlling the spread of diseases while well sited pit latrines do not serve as "seeding bays" for water sources and children paly areas. The proper mix of facilities on an estate save commuting costs for other essentials while an adequate flow of traffic within residences help minimize accidents. Cheap traditional building materials are desired for cost savings. They have implicit health hazards. Thatch roofing imposes danger in fire outbreaks, while mud walling encourages Chagas' disease transmission (Stephens et al; 1985). Traditional wall and floor polishes made from herbs and cow/goat dungs also help to aid worm infestation. The study tests the presence and validity of assertions and linkages for a tropical city using Abeokuta as a case study.

Methodology

The primary data on which most of the analyses in this paper are based are obtained from the results of questionnaire administered on household heads in their dwelling places. Choice of households have been guided by the evolutionary trends of Abeokuta and the variety of housing sub-markets available.

A study of the data on evolutionary trends of Abeokuta reveal three civilizations to which the housing submarkets can be easily tied. These are the early civilization inner core settlements built round the early townships of Ijaiye, Kugba, Alatishe, Igbore, Adatan and parts of Ibara. Hereafter lies the transition areas and the recent Government and suburban residential developments. (Fig. 9.1) The three identified residential strata were subdivided into equal grids using the Abeokuta basemap. A sample size of 10% was aimed at over the city, while the Table of Random Numbers was used to guide chosen study areas. Pilot survey and actual field work was done in the study grid areas.

The pilot survey puts housing estimates at 1448, 1527 and 11550 for the grids in the inner core area, transition area and the Government/suburban areas respectively. Table 9.1 shows the estimated number of houses in each zone and the sample frame.

Table 9.1
Sample frame in study areas

	Estimated No. of Houses	Expected Response	Reliable Response
Core residential area	1448	145	112
Transition district	1527	153	142
Suburban area	1550	155	150
Total	4525	453	404

Source: Authors' Field Survey, 1988.

With a sampling fraction of 1/10, 145, 153 and 155 questionnaires were administered respectively (see Table 9.1 above). However, only 404 questionnaires were properly completed thus giving a 89.18% response to the expected.

The questionnaire used was designed to catch and reflect the epidemiology of some housing related diseases.

Research findings

One major finding of the study which has tremendous influences on other facets of the study is that Abeokuta, is a government workers' town with over 51% of respondents working in government establishments. The employment structure of household heads, for example, show that 49.1% of core-area residents and 52.82% and 53.33% of transition and suburban areas respectively are government worker. The majority of the self-employed as revealed in Table 9.2 exist to service these government institutions and their workers.

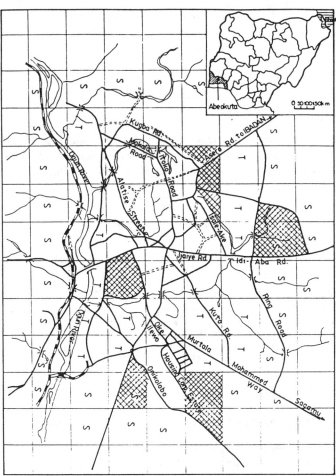

Figure 9.1   Map showing grids and study areas (shaded) of the suburban (S) and transitional (T) areas

From the above observation, it could be inferred that most of the workers are either accommodated in government quarters or given rent allowances to cushion the effects of housing expenditure.

Table 9.2
Employment structure of household heads

	Core Area	Transition Area	Suburban Area
Unemployed	0.00	0.00	0.00
Self-employed	37.5%	35.21%	32.67%
Govt-employed	49.1%	52.82%	53.33%
Retired	13.4%	11.97%	14.00%
Total	100.0%	100.0%	100.0%

Source: Authors' Field Survey, 1988.

Since most of them are literate, there is an observed inkling for adequate housing maintenance especially in the transition and suburban areas. Most of the houses in Abeokuta are however owner occupiers as shown in Table 9.3. This has implications for disease pattern and eventual control.

Table 9.3
Residential status

Status	Core Area	Transition Area	Suburban Area
Owner occupier	34.82%	66.20%	52.67%
Rental-Govt. qtrs	1.78%	2.11%	34.00%
Rental private flats	30.36%	20.42%	9.33%
Rental rooming units	33.04%	11.27%	4.00%
Total	100.0%	100.0%	100.00%
Occupancy ratio	2.80	1.06	1.96

Source: Authors' Field Survey, 1988.

Residential status, residential characteristics and disease ecology

The majority of people in the core area are renters of different sorts and occupying different types of houses (Table 9.3). In the transition and suburban areas, home-ownership predominates. This also has implications for housing maintenance. Existing literature on housing maintenance find positive relationship between high maintenance level and home ownership as opposed to rentals (Labeodan, 1986). It could be inferred that housing maintenance in the core area will be poor or inadequate. This, coupled with its relatively high occupancy ratio of 2.8 (as compared with 1.65 and 1.96 in the transition and suburban zones) call for a close surveillance to stem the potency of any epidemic outbreak.

This possibility becomes more likely when the housing characteristics of the three areas are analyzed. As shown in Table 9.4, over 70% of houses in the core area are rooming houses which not only house a large number of families/people but also exerts enormous pressure on the existing fragile in-house facilities. The type of houses which allows for greater comfort decreases from the core to the periphery. The structural attributes of houses in the different sections of the town show the disease or epidemic prone areas. For example, and a shown in Table 9.5, a significant percentage (35.90%) of houses in the core area are not only old (over 30 years old), but probably due to the traditional mode of design and construction, 33% of them are also poorly ventilated while 14.29% have either unpaved or unbroken floors. This contrasts with findings in the other two sectors. These have a lot of implications for various health risks.

Similarly, different sectors of the town use the open spaces around the house in different ways as this has significant inferences for the spread of diseases. Only 4.93% of people in the transition area use open spaces as dunghill, but in the core area, 8.04% use it as dunghill, 12.50% use it as public toilet and another 59.82% use it for cooking and planting Table 9.6 (see the corresponding figures for other areas). Since these uses are not mutually exclusive, it is probable that as someone is stooling, cooking might be progressing, thus allowing the contamination of the food by diseases carrying flies/insects.

Tenement characteristics and vectors distribution

The different residential peculiarities of each area in the town have wide ranging implications for the presence of vectors in each zone. Table 9.7

Table 9.4
Percentage housing types in the districts

Type	Core area	Transition area	Suburban area
Rooming house	71.43 (80)	44.36 (65)	37.34 (56)
Semi-detached	1.79(2)	1.41(2)	1.79 (2)
Bungalow/flats	9.82(11)	16.20(23)	35.33(53)
Storey blds	16.92(19)	38.03(54)	26.00(39)
Total	100.00 (112)	100.0 (142)	100.0(150.0)

Source: Authors' Field Survey, 1988.

shows the communality of mosquitoes and flies in the three zones and even a decrease of these in the core area (compared with the other two). The core area, however, has an amazing number of mites, ticks, and rats. This shows that the diseases associated with these vectors will be abundantly present in the core area.

Residential districts and disease patterns

Although this research result shows that different types of diseases occur and across the cityscape, their occurrence cannot be said to be district specific (Table 9.8). The study however, found that incidence of a disease is a function of house type occupied. The near uniformity of occupancy ratios subjects the residents of the town to an almost uniform potency of urban health problems. The tendency is, however, greater with the core area residents.

Table 9.5
Structural characteristics of housing in Abeokuta

Variables	Core area	Transition area	Suburban area
Walling			
Plastered	58.04	91.55	90.7
Burnt bricks	5.36	8.45	9.3
Mud walling	36.60	0.00	0.00
Total	100.00	100.00	100.00
Roofing:			
Effective	98.22	100.00	100.00
Defective	1.78	0.00	0.00
Total	100.00	100.00	100.00
Flooring			
Unpaved	8.04	0.00	0.00
Paved & broken	6.25	4.93	4.67
Paved	85.71	95.07	95.33
Total	100.00	100.00	100.00
Age (years)			
Less than 10	10.70	52.10	46.67
$10 < Age < 20$	24.80	32.40	40.00
$21 < Age < 30$	28.60	7.00	13.33
Age > 30	35.90	8.50	0.00
Total	100.00	100.00	100.00

Source: Authors' Field Survey, 1988.

If Table 9.8 is, however, subjected to a comparative analysis on residential district bases, there is a dominance of malaria in all districts. intestinal diseases or disorders like diarrhoea, dysentery and worms are very common in the core area essentially because of the way people lived too close to each other and the way they use open spaces around the house which allows flies fresh from stools to infect food items. The incidence of jigger seems to be localized to the core area too and this may be due to uncemented play areas seeded with various stages of parasites while bare footed children come in contact with these stages in the course of their daily activities.

Table 9.6
Use of spaces around houses

Use of space	Core Area	Transition Area	Suburban Area
Dunghill	8.04	4.93	6.00
& Pub. Toilet	12.50	7.04	10.50
Cooking/Play	59.82	33.10	38.67
Lawns	19.64	54.93	55.33
Total	100.00	100.00	100.00

Source: Authors' Field Survey, 1988.

Table 9.7
Vector around housing units

Vectors	No	Core Res. %	No	Transition Res.	%	Suburban
Mosquitoes, Flies	110	98.2	135	95.07	150	100.00
Mites, ticks	63	56.25	4	2.82	8	5.33
Rats	87	77.68	54	38.03	41	27.33
Snakes, Scorpions	12	10.71	16	11.27	11	7.33

Rs. % Percentage response

Source: Authors' Field Survey, 1988.

Conclusion and recommendations

The general importance of vectors in the ecological system of disease transmission imposed a statistical test to analyze the variance of vectors over the city. Responses on diseases suffered was tested also for its spatial spread across the districts. The F-test was done. The statistical decision imposed is that the differential susceptibility to vectors over the urban space be rejected. This implies homogeneity to certain extent in the properties occasioning vector spread hence disease transmission. Abeokuta is therefore not sufficiently spatially differentiated to allow for localized effects of particular vectors or the diseases they cause.

Table 9.8
Percentage responses to some diseases

Diseases	Core area		Transition area		Suburban area	
	N	%	N	%	N	%
Malaria	112	100	141	99.3	148	98.67
Diarrhoea	78	69.64	11	7.75	3	2.00
Dysentery	101	90.18	39	27.46	8	5.33
Worms	58	51.79	13	9.15	6	4.00
Accidental falls	15	13.39	18	1.68	19	12.67
Jigger	75	64.29	2	1.41	1	0.67
Eczema	18	16.07	21	14.79	13	8.67

Source: Authors' Field Survey, 1988.

Response for certain diseases suffered was tested for spatial effect on its spread. The statistical decision imposed is that district effect is not significant on diseases suffered. However, a test on housing types (tenement surrogate) imposes the rejection of the null hypothesis. This implies that housing type influences accommodation of vectors, hence, also diseases suffered and incidences, irrespective of district location of the house. It could be concluded therefore that based on this research, diseases do not vary across residential districts but across tenement characteristics.

The overall presence of vectors call for wire meshing of windows while environmental sanitation (currently a monthly exercise in Nigeria) need be pursued with all vigour. Households using brooks and wells as water source need to use clean scoops and clean storage pots. Wells too need to be lined and the top made safe against surface inflow and accidental falls. Leaking and defective roofs especially in the core area need to be repaired while poorly ventilated houses may enlarge their windows. Various financial sources are to be relied upon for these remedies while adequate maintenance culture need be encouraged. Socio-cultural enhancement need be encouraged too as a poor blend of these with the most indigenous housing types will readily breed vectors and diseases.

References

Agbola, Tunde (1989). 'The Impact of Urbanization of the Health of Urban Nigerians' in Salem G. et Jeannee, E.(eds.) *Urbanization et. Sante Fanas Le Tiers Monde*, ORSTOM, Paris, pp. 39-60.

Adesina, H.O. (1986). 'Urban Environment and Epidemic Disease', in Adeniyi and Bello-Imam (eds.), *Development and the Environment - Proceedings of a National Conference*, NISER, Ibadan.

Akinbamijo, O.A. (1988). Housing and Health: A Study of the Residential Districts of Abeokuta, *Unpublished Dissertation*, Master in Urban and Regional Planning, University of Ibadan.

Awotona, H.A. (1980). 'Environmental Health Aspects of Housing Nigerians: A Systematic Analysis of Research Needs', *Journal of the Institute of Architects*, June, pp.13-17.

Benevolo, Leonardo (1980). *The Origins of Modern Town Planning*, The M.I.T. Press.

Briscoe, J. and Porter, M. (1987). 'Health and Habitat: The Urban Dimension', *International Planned Parenthood Federation (PPF) Review of Population and Development*, vol. 14, No. 2, pp. 3-5.

Burns, L.S. (1970). *Housing: Symbol and Shelter*, University of California, Los Angeles.

Calhoun, J.B. (1962). 'Population Density and Social Pathology', *Scientific American*, Vol. 206, pp. 139-148.

Chadwick, Edwin (1842). cited in Macpherson (1979),

Clark, R.M. (1978). *An Analysis of Solid Waste, Services: A Systems Approach*, Ann Arbor Science Publishers Inc., U.S.A.

Dunlop, James (1980). 'A Doctor Looks at Housing'. *Housing: The Journal of the Institute of Housing*, vol. 16, No. 3, pp.13-18.

Duvall and Booth, A. (1978). 'Housing and Women's Health'. *Journal of Health and Social Behaviour*, vol. 19, No. 4, pp. 410-417.

Paris and Durnham (1939). cited in Tsung-Yi-Lin (1959).

Galle, O., Gove, R. and Macpherson, J. (1972). 'Population Density and Pathology: What relationships for Man?' *Journal of Health and Social Behaviour*, vol. 14, pp. 209-320.

Gillis, A.R. (1977). 'High-rise Housing and Psychological Strain'. *Journal of Health and Social Behaviour,* Vol. 18, pp. 418-431.

Hardoy, J.E. and Satterthwaite, D. (1987). 'Housing and Health - Do Architect and Planners have a role?' *Cities*, August; Butterworth and Co. (Publishers) Ltd., p. 221-235.

International Year of Shelter and Housing Publication (1987) "Housing on the Brink? *WHO Publication*, Geneva.

Johnson, S. (1897). *The History of the Yorubas*, C.S.S. Press, Lagos.

Kasl and Harburg (1975). 'Mental Health and the Urban Environment: Some Doubts and Second Thoughts', *Journal of Health and Social Behaviour,* vol. 16, pp. 268-282.

Kleevens, J.W.L. (1983). *Housing and Health in a Tropical City: A Selective Study in Singapore*, Assen, The Netherlands, Van Gorcum and Company.

Macleod, S. (1972). 'Environmental Costs and Priorities. A Study at Different Locations and Stages of Development'. *Development and Environment*, UN Conference, Switzerland.

Macpherson, R. (1979). 'Housing and Health: Some Basic Principles' in Murison, H. and Lea, P. (eds.) *Housing in the Third World Countries: Perspectives on Policy and Practice*, Macmillan Press Ltd., pp. 67-82.

Odongo, J. (1978). 'Housing Deficits in Cities of the Third World: Fact or Fiction?' in Murison and Lea (eds.). *Housing in the Third World Countries Perspectives on Policy and Practice*, Macmillan Press Ltd., Hong Kong.

Olaore, G.O. (1987). 'The Cultural Basis of our Environmental Crisis in Nigeria', in Adeniyi and Bello-Imam (eds.) NISER, Ibadan.

Onibokun, A.G. (1986). Two Decades of Public Housing in Nigeria, NISER, Ibadan.

Roberts, B. (1980). 'Home Accidents Related to Personal Safety - A Modern Environmental Health Problems', *Environmental Health*, pp. 142-165.

Sjoberg, G. (1965). 'The Origin and Evolution of Cities'. *Scientific American*, Vol. 213, No. 3, pp. 305-338.

Sommer, R. (1966). 'Man's Proximate Environment': *Journal of Social Issues*, vol. 22, pp. 59-70.

Stephens, B., Mason, J.P. and Isely, R. (1985). 'Health and Low-Cost Housing', *World Health Forum*, Vol. 6, No. 1, pp. 62-69.

Strahler, A. and Strahler, A. (1977). *Geography and Man's Environment*, John Wiley and Sons, New York.

Tipple, A. and Helen, J. (1986). "Priorities for Public Utilities and Housing Improvement in Kumasi, Ghana: An Empirical Assessment Based on Six Variables", *Seminar Paper No. 44*, Univ. of New Castle-Upon-Tyne

Tipple, A.G., Hellen, J.A. and Punce, M.A. (1991). Environmental Risk Assessment in a Tropical City: An Application of Housing and Household Data from Kumasi, Ghana, in Hinz, E. (Editor) *Geonedizinische and biographische Aspekte der Krankheitsverbrieting and Gesundhertsversorgung in Industrie-and Entwicklungstandern* pp. 41-69.

Tsung-Yi-Lin (1959). 'Effects of Urbanization of Mental Health', *International Social Science Journal*, vol. XI, No. 1, pp.110-148.

Wakely, P. J. (1986). "The Devolution of Housing Production support and Management" *Habitat International*, 10, (3) 53-63.

Wirth, L. (1938). 'Urbanism as a way of Life', *American Journal of Sociology*, vol. 44, July, pp. 1-44.

WHO (1961). 'First Report on the Expert Committee on Public Health Aspects of Housing', Report No. 225, Geneva.

WHO (1987). Health in Low Income Communities, *Offset Report*, No.100.

10 Transportation and health in the context of sustainable development: The Nigerian case

Olabode O. Alokan

Summary

This paper examines the environmental and health consequences of transportation activities and discusses the options available for mitigating these within the context of developing countries, using Nigeria as an example. In Nigeria, the health hazards of transportation have had a marked bearing upon the shape of the economy. Until the eighties, road accidents were the major health hazard, but with the onset of recession in the mid-eighties, and the attendant decline in the motorization rate, road accidents too experienced a decline. Nevertheless, the transportation sector in Nigeria is worsening in performance due to the downturn in the economy. The decline in motorization and accident rates has been attended by another hazard in the form of environmental pollution. Although the high traffic volumes of the oil boom era had its attendant air and noise pollution effects, the current decline in the stock of cars and trucks in the country, together with the importation of well-used cars and the poorly maintained public service vehicles, do greater damage to the environment. It is recommended that current efforts at promoting mass transportation in the country should be sustained, to reduce congestion, together with strict enforcement of maintenance regulation and public enlightenment in respect of the environmental consequences of transportation.

Introduction

The derived nature of the demand for transportation implies that there is a definite relationship between transportation and level of development, such that transport infrastructure and activities more or less increase in sophistication with the development of industry and commerce. The transportation industry is better known as the mover of the economy in general rather than a contributor to health problems and environmental stress. But there can be little doubt that the health effects of transportation have a bearing upon economic development. Thus, although the exact nature of the goals of transportation policy varies across countries, the objective of maximizing the contribution of transportation to the national economy, while limiting its adverse effects on the environment, with its obvious consequences for human health, should be central.

Review of health effects of transportation activities

The health hazards of transportation activities are many which for our present purposes, we may categorize into two: 'incidental' and 'general'. Incidental hazard refer to the direct health consequences of using transport facilities by passengers while the 'general' hazards pertain to the general effect of transportation on the environment and, ultimately, on the health status of man. Examples of incidental hazards include (i) malfunctioning of transport equipment (such as a burst tyre) which may lead to fright or shock; (ii) splashing of freight in a moving truck which can cause injury; (iii) a bumpy ride to a hospital which aggravates a patient's illness; (iv) individual personal habits (such as smoking) of passengers who 'force' other to share in the habit; (v) injury arising from badly damaged vehicle seats or from rushing to board a vehicle; and (vi) the tension and anxiety arising from traffic hold-ups. Generally, the continual efforts by vehicle manufacturers to improve upon their products, together with a well coordinated transport sector, will reduce these incidental hazards.

The health hazards of transportation that have gained the forefront in the minds of environmentalists are the atmospheric and noise pollution. The incidence of these latter category of health problems varies across the different transportation media. Also, while some problems cut across all the modes, some are peculiar to some modes.

Table 10.1 sets out the various harmful effects of the various types of particulate matter and gaseous pollutants. Apart from the broader environmental impact of transport and the effects of vehicle emissions on the atmosphere, there are health-related problems that arise from transportation. For instance, it has been argued that "rising levels of a range of gases are altering the thermal structure of the earth's atmosphere and threatening to cause significant changes to the world climate" (Barry and Chorley, 1976). Vehicle emissions are a major contributor to the "Greenhouse" effect and that contribution appears to be increasing (Conlon, 1991).

Water pollution through transportation is largely of the chemical category, and arises basically from the washout of air pollutants produced by fuel combustion (Strahler and Strahler, 1977). Effluents from vehicle garages and auto repair shops can also be washed into drains or directly into streams, but because surface water is normally treated before human consumption, water pollution may not be very serious - at least the amount that can be traced to transportation activities.

Noise is generated by moving traffic and in transport hubs for take-off and landing of equipment. If sufficiently loud, noise may adversely affect people in a number of ways.

Table 10.1
Air pollution effects of transportation activities

Pollutants	Health hazards
Suspended particulate matter (as in smoke, fog, haze, smog)	For persons suffering from respiratory ailments, such as bronchitis and emphysema, the breathing of heavily polluted air can bring on disability and even death.
Carbon monoxide	Death, resulting from interference with the capacity to transport oxygen to the blood.
Oxone	Lethal in large concentrations; eye irritation and possible impairment of lung functions in persons with chronic pulmonary disease; damage to vegetation.
Nitrogen Dioxide	Eye and lung irritant when present in sufficient quantities.
Sulphur Dioxide and Hydrocarbon compounds	When altered by photochemical reaction to produce sulphuric acid and ethylene, respectively, are irritants to the eyes and to the respiratory system; may predispose to the onset of cancer.

Sources: (1) Adapted from Strahler, A.H. and A.N. Strahler (1977); *Geography and Man's Environment*, John Wiley, New York. pp. 56 & 57.

(2) Hobbs, F.D. (1979) *Traffic Planning and Engineering*, Pergamon press, Oxford. pp. 248-250.

Table 10.2 summarizes the effects of noise on humans and gives some examples of sources of various noise levels. In situations (such as happens when operating costs increase substantially) where necessary maintenance is avoided by transport operators, the noise from worn out engines and faulty and unsilenced exhaust pipes can be very serious, apart from the obvious air pollution effect.

Aside from air and noise pollution, other health hazards of transportation include vibrations from moving traffic and severance of people due to the division of an area by roads and traffic, making it difficult, say, to cross heavy streams of traffic and causing not only danger but also delay.

Transport for the disabled and the elderly

Disability and old age do lead people to suffer varying degrees of mobility deprivation. Disability comes in various forms which include sensory impairment (being blind or deaf), intellectual handicap, and physical disability such that people cannot walk very fast or climb steps and kerbs. The needs of people with mobility problems need to be recognized and met. In the United Kingdom, for example, the measures which have been adopted to enable elderly and disabled people and others with mobility problems to use buses more readily include: reduced step heights, low floor buses, additional stanchions and hand-holds and wheelchair access. A low floor bus enables all passengers to board

Table 10.2
Effects of noise and examples of noise levels

Noise effects	Decibels	Typical Examples
Blast deafness	150	Explosions
Pain	140	Engine tests
Threshold of feeling	120	
	110	Thunder, gun fire, Pneumatic drill, aeroplane
	100	
Reduced working efficiency		Underground railway
	90	Busy street
Occupational deafness	85	
		Noisy factory
	80	
Interference with normal Speech		
	70	Noisy office;suburban train
	65	
Annoyance		Factory
	60	
Typing office		Large shop
Restaurant or general Office	50	Quiet office; average house
Private office	45	
Lecture room and suburban living room	40	
Suburban bedroom and library	30	Country road; quiet conversation,whisper
	20	
Very faint	10	Quiet church; sound-proof room. Threshold of hearing

Source: Hobbs (1979), p. 242.

and alight more quickly, so that even though wheel chair users may be carried, running times are not significantly extended.

There are several obstacles to the adoption of these features in a developing country, including that of technology and area-specific problems. In respect of the former, lack of the basic capacity to manufacture and the high cost of custom-built vehicles preclude their wide adoption. As regards the latter, flow-floor buses are unsuitable for rugged terrain and "adverse" road and climatic conditions in developing countries (Barrett, 1989). Besides, the higher demand for public transport in developing countries, much of which is unsatisfied, leaves little consideration for any special provision for disabled persons (Heraty, 1990).

Transport and health problems in Nigeria

Traffic accidents resulting in injury and death undoubtedly rank highest among the health hazards of transportation, especially in Nigeria where it is very serious (Onakomaiya, 1978). However, since 1983, which coincides roughly with the onset of the present economic recession, there has been a steady decline of motorization and with it a gradual drop in the number of road traffic accidents, from 37,000 in 1982 to 26,000 in 1987 and the number of fatalities from 10,367 in 1983 to 7,912 in 1987 (Onakomaiya, 1991). Thus, the general reduction in affluence has been manifested in the progressively lower rates of traffic accidents. The economic crisis has, however, brought to the fore another kind of transport-related health hazards, that of atmosphere and noise pollution and given the prevailing economic situation, this problem will likely become more serious in the years ahead. This is in spite of the fact that pollutants hardly concentrate in the atmosphere in levels high enough to become lethal, and water is normally treated prior to human consumption thus reducing the negative effects of its pollution by transport-generated effluents.

Indeed, from available studies, notably Oluwande (1977), and indirectly from studies of transportation problems by Ogunsanya (1984), Ajai (1983) and Agubamah (1981), the level of pollution is fairly high when compared with other countries. Oluwande's study has shown, for example, that 90% of air pollution problem in Nigeria results from automobile exhaust and that the levels of pollutants such as sulphur dioxide, carbon monoxide and suspended particulate matters, in Ibadan, Nigeria are higher than the World Health Organization's recommended long term limits (see Table 10.3). Furthermore, the concentration of sulphur dioxide in urban areas is about three hundred times the highest in rural areas. Thus, the health effects of air pollution resulting from automobile exhaust is serious in Nigeria, and, as Oluwande has succinctly put it (1977; p. 197 and 198).

> In the major towns ... because of the tropical nature of the climatic condition, many activities are performed outdoors. People stay along the busy roads everyday either to do their work or to sell their wares. The health effects of air pollution resulting from automobile exhaust must be very serious indeed.

This situation is indeed reinforced by the downturn in the economy. The explanation for the air pollution levels experienced in Nigeria in the past was given in terms of (i) the large volume of motor traffic not matched by the rate of highway development; that is, increase in affluence is reflected in more and more vehicles on the road; (ii) the bad state of many of the roads; and (iii) low driving standard of drivers which results in massive traffic hold-up of the kind experienced in western societies with far higher motor traffic volumes.

Table 10.3

Level of pollutants in Ibadan, Nigeria, compared with WHO-recommended long-term limits

Pollutants	WHO limits	Ibadan levels
Sulphur Dioxide	Annual mean: 0.021 ppm. 98% of observation to be below 0.07 ppm.	Annual mean: 0.095 ppm. 40% of observation are below 0.07 ppm.
Carbon Dioxide	8-hour average: 8.6 ppm; 1-hour observation to be below 33 ppm.	Daily average: 7.1 ppm maximum daily average 99.6 ppm.
Particulate and Suspended Matters	Annual mean: 40 mg/m^3. 98% of observations below 120 mg^3/m^3	Annual mean 70 mg/m3 100% observation are below 120 mg^3/m^3

Source: Oluwande (1977, p. 202).

Recent trends in the economy and in the transportation sector bring to the fore the dilemma facing transport administrators, which we may put in the following manner: mobility is imperative for development and the demand for public transport is higher than ever, but the economic crunch largely precludes or limits the acquisition of (new) pollution efficient transport equipment, either for private use or as public service vehicles. Thus, the populace has resorted to (old or fairly used) pollution-intensive equipment, without which mobility would come to a halt. The result of course is a rise in pollution levels. To this extent, sustainable development is being mitigated by economic and fiscal imperatives.

Without any doubt, the volume of traffic in Nigeria has reduced drastically, starting from the early eighties. The national vehicle fleet decreased from over 600,000 in 1982 to about 460,000 in 1988 and to about 300,000 in 1990 (Table 10.4). In addition, newly registered vehicles decreased from over 200,000 (or about 33% of total fleet) in 1982 to 60,000 or 10% in 1986 and to 40,000 or 8.5% in 1988. The decline in the number of new vehicles

114

has been attended by an increase in the number of used cars notably from Western Europe, at a scale of between 10,000 and 20,000 annually. Indeed, a recent report (*The Punch*, 15 January, 1992) has it that imported vehicles account for over eighty per cent of the nation's automobile market, with second-hand vehicles controlling more than seventy per cent of the total vehicle importation. Thus, we have a situation where an estimated 80% of the motor fleet in Nigeria are second-hand, many of which arrive at the ports in a very poor state. The importation has been extended to refurbished engines and other spare parts.

Table 10.4
Motor vehicle fleet in Nigeria

Year	Total vehicles	New registrations	% of Total fleet
1976	197,298	75,000	38.0
1977	224,383	90,000	34.0
1978	260,595	105,000	35.0
1979	295,402	135,000	32.0
1980	357,708	175,000	38.0
1981	428,607	200,000	37.0
1982	504,992	240.000	34.0
1983	599,145	138,000	32.0
1984	614,556	120,000	19.0
1985	607,528	100,000	16.0
1986	602,120	56,000	9.3
1987	547,946	47,000	8.6
1988	466,875	40,000	8.5
1989	385,948	56,000	14.8
1990	302,572	60,000	20.0
1991	350,000	75,000	21.0
1992	280,000	90.000	32.0

Notes: 1. 1988-92 figures are estimates by the World Bank Urban Study Mission to Nigeria, March 1990.

2. A substantial proportion of new registrations since 1988 are of imported used vehicles.

Source: Bolade, A.T. (1991, p. 4)

There are at least two implications of this trend: (i) although traffic volumes have decreased, the resultant pollution generated by the relatively few vehicles on the road is higher than in the past when motorization rate was high, and (ii) even though second-hand vehicles and spares have literally flooded the market, vehicle ownership remains practically an elite preserve, when we consider that the average price of the cheapest of these cars is about thirty thousand naira, as at January, 1992. Thus, the majority of the population bears the cost of mobility of a few. In a period of recession and economic hardship, this additional social cost of transportation is serious. Against the backdrop of recent events in the economy and the transportation scene in Nigeria, it is instructive therefore to examine government policy response to the whole question of the health effects of transportation.

Environmental protection policy in Nigeria

Serious intention by the government to protect the environment in Nigeria is evident in its setting up of the Federal Environmental Protection Agency (FEPA) in 1989. Before that year, probably the only document on the position of government was the publication of the Federal Ministry of Housing and Environment on *The State of the Environment in Nigeria* in 1981. And very recently, the government has come out with the *National Policy on the Environment (NPE)*. *The policy is one that ensures sustainable development based on proper management of the environment in order to meet the needs of the present and future generations.*

Specifically, in respect of air pollution, the NPE has the following strategies for achieving a clean air situation (p. 16 and 17, emphasis mine):

(i)   designating and mapping of National Air Control Zone (ACZ);

(ii)   declaring air quality objectives for each Air Control Zone;

(iii) establishing ambient air quality standards and monitoring stations at each designated zone;

(iv) provision of standards for factories and other activities which emit pollutants into the air;

(v)   provision of guidelines for the abatement of air pollution;

(vi) licensing and registering of all major industrial air polluters and monitoring their compliance with laid down standards;

(vii) prescribing stringent standards for the level of emission from automobile exhausts, and energy-generating plants at stations;

(viii) setting up standards to minimise the *occurrence of "acid rains"*; and

(ix) promoting regional cooperation aimed at minimising the atmospheric transportation of pollutants across international boundaries.

The policy also recognises the need to control noise pollution:
the reduction of noise levels and the control of noise pollution constitute targets for the creation and maintenance of a comfortable and healthy environment. In furtherance of these objectives, programmes will be established to:

(a)   set up noise standards including acoustic guarantees;

(b)   prescribe guidelines for the control of neighbourhood noises especially with respect to construction sites, market and meeting places;

(c)   prescribe permissible noise levels in noise-prone industries and construction sites and to ensure the installation of noise dampers on noisy equipment;

(d)   set up quiet zones especially within game parks, reserves and recreational centres;

(e) provide guidelines for the control of aircraft noise by prescribing acceptable or permissible noise levels within the vicinity of airports;

(f) ensure compliance with stipulated standards by conducting periodic audit checks.

It is clear from these objectives and strategies that the government is not unmindful of both air and noise pollution arising from transportation activities. The policy is, however, not explicit on how to curb air pollution from transportation although it supports prescribing "stringent standards" for the level of emission of automobile exhaust and would "provide guidelines for control of aircraft noise." Nevertheless, the Federal Road Safety Commission (FRSC) has issued a directive making it mandatory for all vehicle importers to obtain road-worthiness certificate *in the country of purchase*, on all second hand vehicles imported into the country.

Towards reducing transport-generated pollution in Nigeria

Several measures have been discussed in the literature for combating transport related pollution (see Bish and Nourse, 1977, for a review). These include reduction in traffic congestion and improvements in traffic speed and flow; encouragement of shifts to mass transportation modes and car-pooling; reduction in lead additives to petrol; installation of emission control devices and adoption of noise abatement technology by manufacturers of vehicles (see Table 10.5). Within the Nigerian context, the most realistic options in respect of air pollution are encouragement of mass transportation modes (to improve traffic flow and reduce congestion), enforcement of vehicle maintenance regulations and insistence on motorists using lead-free petrol. Other solutions such as channelling urban development, encouragement of non-motorized transportation and the move to new technology are either of a long-term nature, of limited usefulness or are technically unrealisable now. Studies have also shown that traffic restraint has had limited success in Nigeria (see Ogunsanya, 1984).

Government has heeded the call for "mass movement" modes (Adeniji, 1983) through its Federal Urban Mass Transit Programme (FUMTP) that is being implemented nationwide. However, from available reports on the progress of the FUMTP (See Filani, 1991 and Viashima, 1991), shortage of buses is a major constraint. With many more buses provided, together with fully functional maintenance back-ups, the bus transit vehicles may come to displace the paratransit modes. Even then, this could be far fetched considering the influx of 'fairly used' vehicles into the country. The reduction in motor traffic volumes occasioned by the high cost of new vehicles and which a more vigorous promotion of bus transit would have helped to sustain, is being mitigated by the influx of these well used cars.

In respect of maintenance regulations, there is no gain-saying the fact that they need to be enforced. Ill-maintained vehicles, evidenced by noisy and smoky exhaust pipes and dilapidated interiors should be kept off the streets. Undoubtedly, this would reduce the

117

Table 10.5
Some control measures of the pollution - effect of transportation

Pollution control measures	Examples	Effects
Adoption of emission control Devices	Non-leaded gasoline Modification of internal combustion engines	
Encouragement of non-motorized transportation (the "slow mode")		
Regulation of traffic	Areal licensing; congestion tolls, Odd/ Even number rule; segregated bus-ways. Highway construction	Lower emissions at higher speeds
Move to new technology	Electrically powered vehicles	
Car-pooling and encourage-ment of mass transportation mode	Provide more public vehicles	Reduction of vehi-cles kilometres travelled energy consumption, congestion and pollution
Strict enforcement of mainte-nance regulation, and of licen-sing and operating laws	Prohibit use of poorly maintained vehicles (e.g. those with worn out engines, unsilenced and faulty exhaust pipes)	
Channel urban development to shorten average journey to work	Suburbanization of work places;	
Noise abatement technology	Hush kitting of aircraft; muffling engine sound. Double-glazing of houses	
Noise charges	To induce manufacturers to produce quieter vehicles and aircraft.	

Source: Adapted from Bish and Nourse, 1975. page 366.

118

number of operators on the road considerably, but their place can be taken by mass transit operators, both public and private. Such a step is considered more conductive than outright economic regulation of the industry, in respect of routes, rates, etc. (Bolade, 1985).

The effectiveness of noise abatement measures in Nigeria would depend, in part, on the success achieved in enforcing road safety and vehicle regulations as well as on the willingness of society to resist the noise effects of air transportation. Indeed, people's perception of noise pollution as a health hazard (Akhtar, 1988) matters a great deal in influencing government's decision as to whether, for example, to impose noise charges or compensate people living near airports for the costs of insulating their homes against noise.

Conclusion

Although transportation and all other non-industrial types of pollution are probably not as serious as the industrial, in developing countries, it nevertheless calls for attention. This is because of the health hazards that continued exposure bring. Air and noise pollution from transportation may get worse considering the downturn in the economy which makes it difficult to purchase new vehicles, encourages transport operators to avoid necessary maintenance of their equipment and generally has led to the poor conditions of the few vehicles on the road. There is need to reduce congestion and associated pollution effects, by improving on the present efforts in respect of mass transportation as well as enforcing maintenance and safety regulation. But perhaps, the most important thing that needs to be done now, as a matter of priority, is to sensitize the citizenry as to the health hazards of transportation. This would make government's policy on environmental degradation much easier to implement.

References

Adeniji, K. (1983). 'Urban Development and Public Transport in Nigeria, *Third World Planning Review* 5(4), 383-94.

Agubamah, C.A.T. (1981). 'Lagos Metropolitan Road Congestion: The Nature of the Problem', *Transport Nigeria*, 1(1), 42-44.

Ajai, J.O.P. (1983). 'Analysis and Solution Identification of the Problems of Heavy Vehicles in the Greater Lagos Area', *Transport Nigeria*, (392), 11-18.

Akhtar, R. (1988). 'Perception of Urban Health Hazards: Examples from Lusaka, Zambia, *Intern. J. Environmental Studies*, 31, 167-172.

Barret, I.M.D. (1989). 'Appropriate Bus Design for Developing Countries, *Developing World Transport*. London: Grosvenor Press International pp. 137-141.

Barry, R.G. and R.J. Chorley (1976). *Atmosphere, Weather and Climate*, Methuen and Co.

Bish, R.L. and H.O. Nourse (1975). *Urban Economics and Policy Analysis*, McGraw-Hill, Kogakusha.

Bolade, A.T. (1985). 'Intermodal Freight Split in Nigeria and its Policy Implications,' *Transportation Policy and Decision Making*, 3, 43-60.

Bolade, A.T. (1991). Towards Evolving an Effective National Mass Transit System: Some Conceptual and Practical Issues. Paper presented at FUMTP/Automania/Anamco Nig. Ltd. seminar on *Towards Effective and Safe Mass Transit in Nigeria*, at National Assembly, Tafawa Balewa Square, Lagos, 25th September, 1991.

Conlon, G.T.P. (1991). 'Public Transport: Making a Comeback', *Transport, Magazine of the Chartered Institute of Transport*, 12(3), 79-82.

Federal Government of Nigeria (1981). *The State of the Environment in Nigeria*, Federal Ministry of Housing and Environment, Environmental Planning and Protection Division, Lagos.

Federal Republic of Nigeria (1989). National Policy on the Environment, Federal Environmental Protection Agency, Lagos.

Filani, M.O. (1991). Emerging Experiences of State-Owned Mass Transit Operators: Case Studies from Oyo and Ondo States. Paper presented at the Federal Urban Mass Transit Programme and Automania Nig. Ltd. seminar on *Towards Effective and Safe Mass Transit in Nigeria*, National Assembly, Tafawa Balewa Square, Lagos, 25th September. 1991.

Heraty, M.J. (1990). Helping Mobility-Handicapped People - and Everyone Else, *Developing World Transport*, London: Grosvenor Press International, pp. 287-292.

Hobbs, F.D. (1979). *Traffic Planning and Engineering*, Oxford: Pergamon Press,

Ogunsanya, A. (1984). 'Improving Urban Traffic Flow by Restraint of Traffic: The Case of Lagos, Nigeria', *Transportation*, 12(2), 183-94.

Oluwande, P.A. (1977). 'Automobile Traffic and Air Pollution in a Developing Country: An Example of Affluence-Caused Environmental Problems', *Intern. J. Environmental Studies*, 11, 197-203.

Onakomaiya, S.O. (1978). *Spatio-Temporal Analysis of Road Accidents in Nigeria*, M.Sc. Project Report, University of Birmingham, U.K.

Onakomaiya, S.O. (1991). 'Trends in Nigerian Road Safety and Accident Situation' in Tunji Bolade and Ade A. Ogunsanya (eds.) *Accident Control and Safety Measures in Mass Transit Operations in Nigeria*, Ibadan University Press.

Viashima, I. (1991). 'Emerging Experiences of State-Owned Mass Transit Operations: Case Studies from Benue and Plateau States'. *Towards Effective and Safe Mass Transit in Nigeria.*

World Health Organization (1972). *Health Hazards of the Human Environment*, Geneva.

Part III
CHANGING LIFESTYLES

Introduction

J. Anthony Hellen

The emergence of new problems of health development in the contemporary Third World presents an extraordinarily varied, complex and challenging range of tasks to those who must seek practical solutions from inside and outside the medical and health sciences. Scientific apartheid seems to have given way to inter-disciplinary collaboration within the university community and the major health agencies at all levels, and new approaches and methodologies are urgently needed.

The international community is tasked with managing an increasingly complex global system in which the very processes of "development" have generated unplanned and often ill-understood convergences and interdependences. Nowhere has this been more marked than in the dynamics of human health and disease in the Third World, as "globalization" process, ranging from rapid urbanization and accelerating industrialization to the diffusion of new technologies and Western consumerism, have altered life-styles and triggered the epidemiological transition.

In a paper which singles out cardiovascular diseases in Nigeria, Akinkugbe reviews the "quiet transformation" which is occurring as their prevalence increases. His clinical and epidemiological data will be of particular interest to those concerned with public health responses, and the reports of the National Task Force for the Control of Non-Communicable Diseases, set up in 1991 and mentioned here, seem likely to be a model for other African countries facing similar morbidity shifts. Iyun's paper on cardiac morbidity in Nigeria is based on hospital admission and medical records from four Ibadan hospitals. It is particularly valuable for relating the cardiac patients to their residential addresses in the inner and out city and the suburbs, as well as in the hinterland of Oyo State and beyond, and establishing a link between the most modern areas of Ibadan with the highest risk amongst those over 45 years of age. The implications for the Nigerian health planners are far-reaching in terms of the cost of premature and avoidable mortality among key members of society.

Foggin's paper concerns health status and associated risk factors of sedentary Tibetan farmers and semi-nomadic pastoralists in Mongolia and the initial phase of a comparative research programme begun in 1991. The data collection promises to be particularly difficult, but here any linkages found between changing life-styles, environmental and health care variables and mortality transitions seem likely to have applications to minority groups surviving in the extensive marginal habitats of the developing countries at large.

Geopsychiatry has to date occupied only a small corner of medical geographical research, but Dory's timely consideration of how empirical and theoretical research should develop is a necessary adjunct to an epidemiological transition model which makes provision for growth in the "socio-pathologies" which appear to accompany development and Westernization. There is certainly a dearth of research into the etiology of mental and psychosomatic illness in Third World communities, and the deficit must be made good.

International travel and tourism, and the associated fields of tourist health and medicine, are used in Hellen's chapter to demonstrate the emerging linkages and interdependencies between developed and developing countries represented by the global leisure revolution. The somewhat belated responses by the medical profession and the travel industry to the health implications of these massive transfers of transient tourist populations to tropical and sub-tropical areas are a salutary lesson to those geographers whose expertise in the tropical world has found few applications within the health sector.

Taken together these contributions are to be seen as reflecting interest on the one hand in the "Westernization" of disease and health problems in the developing countries, and on the other in the "tropicalization" of disease risks likely to affect significant sectors of a global tourist industry dominated by markets in the developed countries.

11 Geopsychiatric problems in developing countries

Daniel Dory

Summary

The paper deals with some specificities of geopsychiatric research in developing countries. Mainly the problems of identification and localisation of psychiatric cases, the complexity of the health care resources, (traditional and modern) and the cultural interpretation of mental diseases. After a brief survey of the main trends of current research, some methodological and theoretical perspectives are proposed.

Introduction

Geopsychiatry refers to geographical research concerning both the spatial distribution of mental health problems (in a broad sense), and the territorial organization of diverse mental health care services or structures (Dory, 1991). Geopsychiatry is a new and specialized field in medical geography, having been recognized as a distinct topic in geographic literature for the last two decades. As this field is still in its youth, there remains a lack of unquestionable laws and conclusions. We can confidently argue, nevertheless, that both the empirical materials gathered and the theoretical statements already formulated, permit and call for a more fundamental discussion (Sivadon 1948). Although some researchers find this endeavour useless or even dangerous, we would insist on the fact that without it the risk exists of building a discipline where the answers (even nicely translated into sophisticated mathematical figures) largely outnumber the questions.

These problems of theoretical pertinence are of special relevance in the case of geopsychiatric issues in developing countries, where but for a few exceptions (Sule, 1981), we are facing a dramatic scarcity of research materials. This statement does not imply, however, the assumption that there exists a radically heterogeneous reality distinguishing between "developed" and "developing" countries in the particular field of mental health problems. On the contrary, many indications, (as shown below) tend to confirm the fecundity and the appropriateness of a "continuist" approach. This approach postulates, concerning health problems, that differences should be more efficiently analyzed when viewed in terms of quantitative variation rather than qualitative gaps. This is even more relevant when we consider the enormous differences between countries which are included inside one or another of those large groups; (for instance, China, Burkina Faso, Mexico or Nigeria, are all included in the broad category "developing countries").

This contextual introduction allows us to assert that if the five statements concerning the geopsychiatric approach that we will formulate in this paper are directly relevant to the context of developing countries, they have, nevertheless, a boarder scope. Indeed, we strongly believe that these topics will shape empirical and theoretical research concerning geographical aspects of mental health problems in the next few years. The five points are the following.

Geopsychiatry puts us in a position to consider the maximal, (and not only the minimal) conditions of health status.

In addition to the "classical" and dramatic health problems experienced by developing countries, which can be divided into two (strongly interrelated) broad categories: nutritional deficiencies (culminating or not in famine episodes), and infectious and parasitic diseases (Acuna *et al.* 1981); to argue for special concerns for mental health problems can be, and very frequently is, considered futile or a luxurious waste of scarce resources.

In fact, probably only a very small percentage of persons suffering from a more or less serious psychiatric symptomology, (point prevalence is evaluated by the W.H.O. at an average of 5% of the whole population at a given moment), receives specialized mental health care. This situation with its dramatic individual and collective consequences is also the product of practical and intellectual division of health care services, where somatic and nutritional problems are first considered. In the end, if some money and qualified health care providers remain available, mental health care will retain some attention.

In contrast with this situation, reflected also to some extent in the specialized literature of medical geography, it is useful to emphasize that geopsychiatry makes it possible to contain the basic conditions of human health. These conditions are fundamentally psychosomatic and social as far as health is a function of the relations of individuals and groups, with the enormous diversity of natural and manmade environments. In other words, by studying the environmental conditions of mental health and health care, geopsychiatry allows the general field of medical geography to analyze the complex determinants of a comprehensive definition of human health. In this sense, geopsychiatry also helps the geography of health to cross artificial boundaries between specialized, theoretical and practical fields. In understanding the human subject in natural, historical and cultural environments we will see an individual whose integrity should not be divided (Dreikure, 1953).

In this way, the transition from the study of minimal to maximal (or optimal) sanitary conditions, allows the definition not only of basic survival issues, but more conveniently health status, including all the necessary components of a full human life.

Geopsychiatric research implies the analysis of environments in their whole complexity

This point assumes permanent relations between geopsychiatry on one side and the main trends of current research both in physical and human geography on the other side. Such an uninterrupted dialogue could also help as a reminder that distinctive objects of geographic science are territories and all the specialized fields of geography are supposed to throw some significant light on this topic. This territorial knowledge, which must be developed in an interdisciplinary framework (Gold, 1982) is centred upon two main problems:

(a)　The question of the reactional etiology of mental and psycho-somatic illness, implies the discovery of what exactly in the environment can be pathogenic, for whom, and under which conditions.

(b)　The problem of variation in notoriously pathogenic factors (under some defined conditions) among more or less homogeneous territorial unities in relation with other variables.

For instance, these issues could be explored by a methodical study of a factor, such as the fear of crime. This condition, despite the fact that it is almost never mentioned in the medical geographic literature, has unquestionable impacts on the daily lives of a large proportion of the population (mainly) in large urban centres of developing and developed countries. We also know the differential impact of this pathogenic factor in relation to the localization of individuals, their characteristics (age, sex, former victimization, etc), and the type of crimes to which they are (or believe they are) exposed. These issues should be investigated in collaboration with researchers dealing with the geography of crime (Smith, 1986). But here again we are confronted with a dramatic scarcity of data concerning developing countries. This contrasts with the fact that this part of the world is experiencing an enormous increase in crime rates, connected with uncontrolled population increase, high unemployment, rural-urban migrations, etc. It seems reasonable, nevertheless, at this point to advocate, concerning those matters, that at least as much attention should be given to the victims as to the criminals.

Geopsychiatry invites us to consider individuals in their whole psychosomatic integrity

Again, basic evidence is provided essentially by research conducted in developed countries, but the importance of this item makes it impossible to be omitted.

For instance Vasquez Barquero et al. (1987), in a survey of a broad spectrum of epidemiological literature, arrived at the following quantitative indications, which clearly shows the futility of considering separately somatic or psychiatric troubles:

127

- The proportion of psychiatric patients presenting equally significant somatic illness can be estimated from 33% to 68%.
- On the other hand, among persons affected by severe somatic troubles, symptoms of mental pathology can be as high as 70%, (mainly depression, anxiety, psychotic reactions, etc.).

In the particular context of a rural area in a developing country, (Niakhar in Senegal), Diop et al. (1980) found out from the consultants of a primary health care structure that:

- An average of 17% of patients presented a psychiatric symptomatology among the children between 5 and 15 years, (N = 545).
- More than 16% of the sample of adults asking for health care showed signs of mental health problems, in addition or not to a somatic trouble, (N = 933).

This kind of data should prevent a narrowly conceived approach to health problems, in this field of geography as well as in others. At a more theoretical level the notion of stress could allow the creation of a more comprehensive research framework aimed at consolidating the psychosomatic orientation within medical geography (Hunter, 1974).

Geopsychiatry invites us to overcome some arbitrary partitions in the analysis of health phenomena, and in the study of the relationships between societies and environments.

Two examples illustrate this point.

(a) First, it is necessary to emphasize the imperative of considering both the objective and the perceptive characteristics of environments concerned by sanitary issues (Kellett, 1984). Here again, a double interdisciplinary perspective is useful; simultaneously inside geography also (mainly focused on the relations with sociology and cultural anthropology when dealing with the social determination of the organization and interpretation of environmental significant features). At the moment, however, the basis of a theory that is able to generate non-ethnocentric hypotheses in this field is still lacking.

(b) Secondly, there is a real need to fill a somewhat artificial and largely non-existent gap in developing countries. This gap exists between the modern/medical/formal mental health sector, and the informal or traditional/popular one. The objective could be reached by a systematic analysis of the individual and collective *therapeutic itineraries* taking into consideration, for each illness episode, all the health care seeking decisions and referrals. The spatial aspect of this issue must also be elucidated by the study of the diversity in health services of all kinds in a given area (Good 1979).

Geopsychiatry invites us to put practical action in a really explicit ethical perspective

This point refers to the full implications of the global definition of health mentioned at the beginning of this paper. This globality includes:

- The whole Planet, whose resources should be managed in a careful way in view of present and future social needs.
- All the aspects of human life in their territorial dimension, and how they are affected by potentially harmful environmental factors.
- The total complexity of an individual's existence.

More generally, and beyond the necessary care to the heaviest psychiatric cases, this approach compels all societies to define optimal environmental mental health conditions: thereby formulating in an explicit form, the conditions of a really human life. This problem is particularly crucial because, if survival implies not being affected by infant mortality, accidents, lethal diseases of the adult period, famine or suicide, all those conditions are not enough to provide an optimal human life. To reach this aim, structured environments, good nutritional conditions, schools, decent employment, good housing, individual and collective security, social solidarities, etc. are essential. It is neither utopic nor unrealistic to remember those elements when thinking about mental health problems in developing countries (OMS/WHO, 1981).

All societies, in relation to their own history and culture have to elaborate this global aims of human life under the form of social optimal projects and ideal goals. This also implies a territorial planning conceived in relation to the lessons of geopsychiatric research, (and more generally with skills in medical geography, which must be promoted by systematic training in as many geography departments as possible (Saenz de la Calzada, 1971). Geographers now have to show both those needs and try to answer the questions they raise. So we are probably at the beginning of an exciting intellectual and practical adventure, on condition, however, that we believe that a worse future is not necessarily inevitable.

References

Acuna, H.R. (1981). 'Health priorities in Latin America and the Pan American Health Organisation', *Social Science and Medicine* Vol. 15D, pp. 537-539.

Carstairs, G.M. (1984). 'Mental health and the environment in developing countries', in Freeman, H.L., ed. *Mental health and the environment*. London, Churchill Livingstone, pp. 425-452.

Diop, B. (1980). *et al.* 'Symptomatologie et diagnostic psychiatriques dans une region rurale du Senegal', *Psychopathologie Africaine*, No 1, pp 5-20.

Dory, D. (1990). 'La geographie de la sante: questions theoriques', *Revue Belge de Geographie*, fasc. 4, pp. 171-179

Dory, D. (1991). *Elements de Geopsychiatrie*, L'Harmattan, Paris.

Dreikurs, R.H. (1953). *Fundamentals of Adlerian Psychology*. Chicago, Alfred Alder Institute.

Eyles, J. (1990) 'How significant are the spatial configurations of health care systems?' *Social Science and Medicine*, Vol. 30, No, pp. 157-164.

Giggs, J.A. (1977). 'Mental disorders and mental subnormality' in Howe, (G.M.), ed. *A World Geography of Human Diseases*. London, Academic Press, 1977. pp. 477-506.

Giggs, J.A. (1980). 'Mental health and the environment' in Howe, (G.M.); Loraine, (J.A.) eds. *Environmental Medicine*, London, Heinemann, (2nd ed.), pp. 281-305.

Giggs, J.A. (1986). 'Ethnic status and mental illness in urban areas', in Rathwell, (T.); Phillips, (D.), eds., *Health, Race and Ethnicity*, London, Croom Helm, pp. 137-174.

Giggs, J. A. (1986) "The Spatial Ecology of Mental Illness" in Smith, S.J. Crime, *Space and Society*, Cambridge, Cambridge University Press.

Gold, J.R. (1982). 'Territoriality and human spatial behaviour', *Progress in Human Geography*. Vol. 6, No 1, pp. 44-67.

Hellen, J.A. (1986). 'Medical geography and the Third World' in Pacione, M., ed. *Medical Geography: Progress and Prospect*. London, Croom Helm, pp. 284-332.

Hunter, J.M. and Brunn, S.D. (1974). 'The geography of psychosocial stress' in Hunter, (J.M.), ed. *The Geography of Health and Disease*. University of North Carolina at Chapel Hill, Studies in Geography No 6, pp. 128-153.

Iyun, F. (1989) 'Some observations on the spatial epidemiology of mental ill-health in Nigerian cities: a preliminary investigation of Ibadan mental clinics', in *Urbanisation et Sante dans le Tiers Monde* ORSTOM, Paris, pp. 61-73.

Kellett, J.M. (1984). 'Crowding and territoriality: a psychiatric view', in Freeman, H.L. ed. *Mental Health and the Environment*. London, Churchill Livingstone, pp. 71-96.

OMS/WHO (1981). *Dimensions sociales de la sante mentale*, Geneve.

OMS/WHO, (1984) *Les soins de sante mentale dans les pays en developpement: bilan critique des resultats et de la recherche*, Geneve,

OMS/WHO, (1988). Huitieme programme general de travail pour la periode 1990-1995; Programme 10, Protection et promotion de la sante mentale, Geneve.

Prothero, R.M. (1963) 'Medical geography in tropical Africa', in McGlashan, (N.D.); Blunden, (J.R.), eds. *Geographical Aspects of Health*, London, Academic Press, 1983, pp. 137-153.

Saenz de la Calzada, C. (1971). 'La information academica del especialista en geografia medica en Mexico', *Annuario de Geografia* (UNAM), pp. 103-105.

Sivadon, P. (1948). 'Geographie humaine et psychiatrie', *Cong. Med. Al. et Neurolog. de Fr.*, Marseille, Masson, Paris pp. 3-48.

Smith, C.J.(1978). The Geography of Mental Health, Association of American Geographers, *Resource Paper* N° 76-4, Washington.

Smith, S.J. (1986) *Crime Space and Society*, Cambridge, Cambridge University Press.

Sule, O.R.A. (1981). 'Spatial patterns of urban mental health: Calabar (Cross River State) Nigeria', *Geojournal* Vol. 5, No. 4, pp. 323-330.

Vasquez-barquero, J.L. (1987). *et al.* 'Salud fisica y enfermedad mental. Un analisis epidemiologico', *Actas Luso-Espanolas de Neurologia, Psiquiatria y Ciencias Afines*, 13/3, pp. 151-163.

Verhasselt, Y. (1987). 'Environmental changes and health in tropical Africa', *Revue Belge de Geographie*, No 3-4, pp. 191-196.

12 Health status and risk factors research in two East Asian populations: Tibetans of western China and the semi-nomadic Herdspeople of Mongolia

Peter M. Foggin

Summary

This paper gives an overview of the theoretical and conceptual model that is at the base of geographical health status and risk factor research, pointing out that health status is largely a function of behavioural factors, environmental conditions and health care system variables. An overview of some general indicators of the health status of the populations of Mongolia and the Tibetan Plateau region of western China form the foundation for research which is in its beginning stages in this part of East Asia. A description is given of the field work that is to be undertaken.

Introduction

Every culture builds a system of beliefs, knowledge and practice in relation to its experiences of life, health and disease - which is the realm of ethnomedicine (Fabrega and Hunter, 1977; Fabrega and Manning, 1979; Mechanic, 1961; Segall, 1976). The syndrome-culture interaction has been emphasized by authors such as Sanders (1964), and traditional medicine itself has a significant impact on this relationship (Arkerknecht, 1942; Stock, 1980). Significantly, the behaviour of patients and health practitioners, as well as the placing of health care in its locational context have been widely studied by geographers (Stock, 1980, 1982, 1983; Shannon and Dever, 1974; Pyle, 1979; Picheral, 1982, 1989). At another level, the social system itself can be viewed as a casual factor related to the incidence of disease, in as much as it is an integral part of the total environment (social-physical-biological) in the so-called epidemiological and ecological host-agent-environment triad (Learmonth, 1978; Meade 1977; Meade *et al*, 1988). These theoretical concerns come into focus through research on the health status and risk factors of two major cultural groupings that have never been systematically studied in this way: the Tibetans of Western China and the semi-nomadic herdspeople of Outer Mongolia.

The high incidence of certain infectious diseases (e.g., acute respiratory infections) and relatively high infant mortality rates are but two of the indicators of a very problematic situation which is found in many of the geographically remote populations of the world. This is particularly true of the two population groups that this study investigates. There is no doubt that better programmes of preventive health care are needed. The practical importance of this research, then, is that of seeking to understand and explain the dynamics and relationships between health status levels and their corresponding risk factors - this knowledge being essential to the formulating of effective and relevant programmes of preventive health care.

The ecological model

This research is more ecological than epidemiological in its approach. By "ecological" is understood the relating of observed levels of health with the various characteristics of the behavioural, social and physical environments. Furthermore, the term "ecological" is used in the sense of an approach where the basic observational unit of analysis is a village, population grouping or any other unit corresponding to a spatial area, rather than an analysis carried out on an individual basis (Briggs and Leonard, 1977; Meade 1977; Meade et al, 1988).

The health status of a minority population (viewed as the "dependent" variable) varies as a function of (1) life-style factors (e.g., diet, tobacco and alcohol consumption, geographic mobility), (2) demographic and socio-economic characteristics (e.g., age, sex, income), (3) the social, physical and medical environments (e.g., family-size quality of drinking water, availability of and accessibility to health care services, respectively) (Fogin and Philie, 1984; Foggin and Lauzon, 1986; Brodman et al, 1954; Daly, 1972; Aurillon, 1987). This hypothesis flows from a multi-dimensional conceptual framework (Anderson et al., 1976, pp. 10-23) where health status is viewed in the context of three broad dimensions: 1) the "natural system", 2) the "social system", and 3) the "psycho-biological" system. The above hypothesis, while majoring on the "natural" (physical environment) and "social" (socio-economic and behavioural factors), also involves the "psycho-biological" at the level of measuring the dependent variable (i.e., health status).

Health status indicators: Tibetans and Mongolians

On the Tibetan side, the high infant mortality rates are commonly associated with acute respiratory infections (ARI) and dehydration due to diarrhoea. With regard to endemic disease, tuberculosis is a major problem. Also noteworthy is the little-understood and frequently mentioned (in Tibetan areas) "big-bone disease" - a deforming illness which in some Tibetan villages affect as many as 50% of the population. Goitre is another endemic disease among Tibetans (Boutriau, 1990). The infant mortality (IM) rates associated with the countries involved in this study's specific Tibetan target population are: Aba county - IM = 156 per thousand; Xiahe county - IM = 64 per thousand; Tongren county - IM = 79 per thousand.

On the Mongolian side, the largest subgroup is the Khalkha, accounting for over 75% of the total population. Migration from rural areas has accelerated with 58% of Mongolians now living in urban areas" (Milne *et al*, 1991, p.2). The cities are surrounded by temporary and make-shift rural dwellings, predominantly ger or "yurts". In rural areas, 50% of the families of farmers and herdsmen live below the level of subsistence. School attendance is compulsory for children 8-15 years, and while official statistics indicate that 100% of the population is literate (WHO., 1991, pp. 4-5), preliminary field work casts doubt on such a figure. IM and U5MR rates have already been discussed. The rate of natural population increase is over 3%.

In Mongolia, the leading causes of mortality in persons of all ages (% of all deaths in hospitals in 1989) are: respiratory diseases = 35.7%; gastrointestinal diseases = 15.5%; heart diseases = 9.3%; perinatal diseases = 9.3%; infectious and parasitic diseases = 8.8%; tumors (neoplasms) = 7.2% (WHO, 1991, p. 6). Leading causes of morbidity follow the same pattern, in so far as respiratory and gastro-intestinal diseases are concerned. ARI and gastroenteritis are the leading causes of morbidity and mortality in children. Meningitis and hepatitis B are showing increasing annual incidence rates (WHO, 1991, p.6).

Conditions of field research

The situations for field work are vastly different for the two population groups. For various reasons it is extremely difficult for an international researcher to carry out social research in the P.R.C. However, since the radical changes that have come about in the M.P.R. since 1990, there is a new openness to effective international cooperation in all areas of scientific endeavour, including social sciences such as medical geography. In fact, it is possible to work in China only under the auspices of a recognized scientific body, and this is what we are doing with the Department of Geography of the Sichuan Normal University. Collecting useful and relevant data in the various counties whose population are predominantly Tibetan is a definite challenge to cultural and medical geographers.

In Mongolia preventive health care and public health have high priority, and there is a general atmosphere of openness to international expertise, all of which contribute to a climate conducive to cooperative research projects such as this one. The senior research team is composed of two Mongolian colleagues (Chinbat of the Geography Department of the Mongolian State University, and Shirev of the Institute of Geography of the Mongolian Academy of Sciences), a Hungarian graduate student (O. Farkas) fluent in Mongolian and English and the author of this paper. Chinbat and Shirev have been working for the past ten years on the ecology/geography of animal husbandry among the nomadic herspeople of Mongolia while Farkas has been studying the Mongolian language and cultures over the past six years. Foggin has been working on the health

135

status and risk factors of the Inuit and Cree of northern Canada for the past ten years, and developing his Asian interest since 1987.

A field trip carried out in October, 1991 in Ovorhangay aimak (province) revealed a great willingness on the part of local populations to be involved in the proposed health status and risk factor survey. The plan is to carry out a first survey in 1992 in three *sumon:* one in the *"hangay"* or wooded mountain steppe where yak husbandry dominates, one on the regular steppe where sheep dominate; and one in the gobi or desert environment where camel husbandry is the central activity. In each of these sumon, each household or *ger (yurt)* is located either alone or in a group of yurts (a *"hotail"*, i.e., from one to ten yurts in a group). Each of these hotail has been located on detailed maps, and has a different location for each of the four seasons. This relatively ordered, nomadic life-style will be systematically documented and related, among other factors, to the health status of each household. In contrast, the Tibetan population of the study counties of Sichuan is composed of sedentary farmers. Here, the people are settled in many small, but permanent, village-hamlets. Each village in the study's random village sample will be studied in its entirety.

Expected results

There are two levels of results that are envisaged: practical and scientific. On the Mongolian side, there is definitely a desire on the part of the government to promote this kind of study with a view to understanding the dynamics of the situation in order to provide more effective programmes of health care. One of the most problematic aspects of health care in Mongolia is the challenge of meeting the health and educational needs of a population which moves seasonally from one location to another, (moves of often over 50 kilometres). The practical applications of this work in the Chinese context are less clear, given the prevailing socio-political context.

At the scientific level it should be remembered that this is a comparative study, measuring the health status and various parameters linking three families of variables to health status (environmental, life-style and health care characteristics) of different, geographically isolated populations. The two new populations studied (Tibetan and Mongolian) will be related to each other and to two populations previously researched: the Inuit and Cree of northern Quebec province in Canada. The literature indicates that health status is broadly related to each of these three bodies of variables. What this study is seeking to do is to describe the shape (i.e., the specific parameters) of these relationships. It is expected that there will be marked similarities between the four population groups, notwithstanding major cultural and geographic difference.

References

Ackerknecht, E.M. (1942). Problems of primitive medicine. *Bulletin of history and medicine* 11: 503-521.

Akinar, A. (ed.) (1991). *Mongolia Today*. London: Kegan Paul.

American Thoracic Society (1978). *Standardized Epidemiological Questionnaire* (including detailed guide).

Anderson, Kohn, R. and White, K.L. (1976). *Health Care: An International Survey.* London: Oxford University Press.

Aurillon, N. (1987). *L'etat de sante des Inuit du Nouveau-Quebec: etude de geographie medicale socio-culturelle.* These de 3ieme cycle Geographie. Universite Paul-Valery, Montpellier.

Banister, J. (1987). *China's Changing Population.* Stanford: Stanford University Pre Asian Studies.

Boutriau, D. (1990). Programme d'appui aux structures de sante de base des Cantons de Lingzhou et Nimou, District de Lhasa, Region autonome du Tibet. Brussels: *Medecins Sans Frontieres:* Project proposal for a 3-year programme in Tibet (1991-1994).

Breymeyer, A. and Klimek, K. (eds) (1983). *Mongolian Dry Steppe Geo-systems.* Warsaw: Ossolineum, The publishing house of the Polish Academy of Sciences.

Briggs and Leonard (1977). Mortality and ecological structure. *Social Science and Medicine* 11D.

Brodman, K., Ersmann, A.J., Wolff, H.G. (1954). *Cornell Medical Index: Health Questionnaire.* Cornell Univ. Medical College.

Chabros, K. (1983). *La nomadisation Mongole: Techniques et Symbolique.* Bloomington: University of Indiana, Research Institute for Inner Asian Studies.

Collective work (1990). *Information Mongolia: Analysis of Census Information.* London: Pergamon Press.

Daly, M.B. (1972). Cornell medical index response as predictor of mortality. Br. *J. of preventive social medicine* 26.

Ekvall, R.B. (1968). *Fields on the hoof: Nexus of Tibetan nomadic pastoralism.* New York: Holt, Rinehart and Winston.

Ekvall, R.B. (1964). *Religious observances in Tibet: Patterns and Functions.* Chicago: University of Chicago Press.

Ekvall, R. B. (1952). *Tibetan Skylines.* New York: Farrar, Straus and Giroux, Inc.

Fabrega, H. Jr. (1974). *Disease and social behaviour; An interdisciplinary perspective. Cambridge*, MA: MIT Press.

Fabrega, H. and Hunter, J.E. (1977). The effects of disease on behaviour. *Ethos* 5: 119-137.

Febrega, H. and Manning, P.K. (1979). Illness episodes, illness severity and treatment options in a pluralistic setting. *Social Science and Medicine* 13B: 41-51.

Feldman, J.J. (1960), The household interview as a technique for the collection of morbidity data. *J. Chron. Disease* 11, p. 535.

Foggin, P.M. and Aurillon, N. (1989). Respiratory health indicators and acculturation among the Inuit and Cree of Northern Quebec. *Social Science and Medicine* 29: 617-626.

Foggin, P. M. and Lauzon, H. (1986). Health Status and Risk Factors: the Cree of Northern Quebec. Dept. de geographie, Univ. de Montreal.

Foggin, P. M. and Philie, P. (1984). Health Status and Risk Factors: the Inuit of Northern Quebec. Dept. de geography, Universite de Montreal.

Lariviere, Jean-Pierre et Sigwalt, Pierre (1991). La Chine. Paris: Masson/Geographie.

Learmonth, A. (1978), *Patterns of Disease and Hunger: A Study in Medical Geography.* London: David and Charles.

Lee, D.H.E. (ed.) (1972). *Environmental Factors in Respiratory Disease.* New York: Academic Press.

Meade, M. (1977). Medical geography as human ecology: the dimension of population movement. *Geographical Review* 67: 379-393.

Meade, M., Florin, J. and Gestler, W. (1988). *Medical Geography.* New York: Guildford Press.

Mechanic, D. (1961), The concept of illness behaviour. *J. Chron. Disease* 15: 189-194.

Milne, E., Leimone, J., Rozwadowski, F. and Sukachevin, P. (1991). Washington, *The Mongolian People's Republic: Toward a Market Economy.* D.C.: International Monetary Fund (April, 1991).

P.O.M.S. (1991). Health Status and Health Care: W.H.O. Programme in Mongolia. Ulaan Baatar, 42 pages.

Picheral, H. (1982). Geographie medicale, geographie des maladies, geographie de la sante. *L'Espace Geographique* 11: 161-175.

Picheral, H. (1989). Geographie de la transition epidemiologique. *Annales de geographie* 98: 129-151.

Pyle, G. (1979). *Applied Medical Geography.* Washington, D.C.: Winston/Wiley.

Segall, A. (1976). Sociocultural variation in sick role behavioural expectations. *Social Science and Medicine* 10: 47-51.

Shannon, G. and Dever, A. (1974). *Health Care Delivery: Spatial Perspectives.* New York: McGraw-Hill.

Stock, R. (1980). Health and health care in Hausaland. In F.A. Barrett (ed.) *Canadian Studies in Medical Geography.* Toronto: York University Geographical Monograph, 190-2.

Stock, R. (1983). Distance and the utilization of health care facilities in Nigeria. *Social Science and Medicine* 17: 563-570.

Thouez, J.P. et Foggin, P.M. (1989). Hypertension et modernite: resultats d'une enquete effectuee chez les Cris et les Inuit du Nord du Quebec. *Le geographe canadien* 3: 18-30.

UNICEF (1990). *An analysis of the situation of children and women in Mongolia - 1990.* Ulaan Baatar: UNICEF.

World Health Organization (1991). *Health Status and Health Care: WHO Programme in Mongolia.* Ulaan Baatar, 42 pages.

13 Cardiac morbidity in Nigerian society: Trends and inter-relationships

B. Folasade Iyun

Summary

The contribution of non-infectious, and in particular cardiac, disease is often compromised by the relatively low rates of reporting in our medical institutions. Even though infectious and parasitic diseases appear to continue to play a prominent role in our morbidity trends, there is some evidence of gradual but significant contributions of non-communicable diseases and especially heart disease in our adults.

This paper attempts to give some credence to the now obvious signs of an epidemiological transition in the Nigerian society. The paper relies on two sets of data:

(i) prospective data of three hospitals' admissions between January 1989 and 31 December, 1990 in Ibadan city;

(ii) retrospective data of total cardiac attendance at the University College Hospital (UCH) from 1957 to 1990.

The results of the data analysis indicate that more men were affected by cardiac disease, and that the fatality rated between 24% and 26%. It was obvious that patients aged 45 years and above were mostly afflicted. There are also indications of more admissions in the month of August.

The spatial distribution of the admissions was also of interest. In the three study hospitals for the prospective data, the outer areas of the city recorded 43% to 83% of all the admission cases. The retrospective data also clearly corroborates the general rise in the trend of cardiac disease and suggests that it is prevalent in the suburbs and among the affluent. The general conclusion is that as we advance in national development, there is the tendency for the well-to-do individuals to carry higher risks of cardiac disease.

In conclusion, in the process of national development the well-to-do appear to be susceptible to cardiac disease. It is therefore imperative for such individuals to undergo regular medical examinations to reduce the incidence of sudden cardiac attacks. In addition, health education is vital in this respect, especially as more of our national population will increasingly move into the most affected age group.

Introduction

The contributions of infectious and parasitic diseases often attract substantial attention in both the medical and biomedical sciences since they frequently provide the most obvious manifestations of the medical environment in the Third World countries. In comparison, the contribution of non-infectious, in particular cardiac diseases are often compromised by the relative low rates of reporting of such diseases in the majority of our medical institutions, with little or no information in such diseases in the official health statistics. Even though infectious and parasitic diseases appear to continue to play a prominent role in our morbidity trends, there is some evidence of gradual but significant contributions of non-communicable diseases, especially heart diseases and other degenerative diseases. Besides this, in recent times, it appears there is an on-going, albeit invisible, epidemiological transition in the Nigerian medical environment, which now fosters an increase in the incidence of non-infectious and parasitic diseases.

This paper attempts to give some credence to the increasing relative importance (perhaps signs of epidemiological transition) of cardiac disease in the Nigerian society which may be representative of what now happens in other African cities. Hence, the paper focuses on the relative importance of the major cardiac conditions and their trends, socio-demographic characteristics of the sufferers and their spatial dimension in the urban setting.

Data and methods

The enormous problem created by the lack of existence of hard data to verify epidemiological transition in Nigeria is fully appreciated. In Nigeria, there is a general lack of systematic reporting and analysis of morbidity data within and among medical institutions and geographical regions. Even though some medical practitioners have provided some important analyses of cardiac disease based on hospital data in some African cities (Edington, 1954, Accra; D'Arbela, 1966, Carlisle and Ogunlesi, 1972, Akinkugbe, 1992, among others), the emphasis has been placed on the relative significance of each condition in terms of level of incidence and the predominance of each disease between the sexes and the different age groups.

The present analysis also has to contend with two sets of data that are hospital-based: (i) prospective data from three major hospitals in Ibadan city and (ii) retrospective data of the University of Ibadan Teaching Hospital (UCH).

The collection of the prospective data from the University College Hospital (UCH), the Oyo State-owned Ring Road State Hospital (RRSH) and the Jericho Nursing Home (JNH) commenced in January 1989 and ended in December 1990. The data consist of admission records at the hospitals' medical wards. At the UCH, the services of a medical record clerk were engaged for the period. He normally was one of those in charge of retrieving admission cases for the Hospital Medical Records Department for compilation. The retrieval of the records was on daily basis, or at the very worst at the end of each week. For the other two hospitals, a trained graduate research assistant visited each hospital at the end of each week to compile the admission cases. The retrospective data were collected from the UCH Medical Records Department. These comprise the total attendance of cardiac patients from 1957 to 1990.

The data collection involved accurate recording of the physicians' diagnosis in the case notes or admission registers. It was not practicable to verify the diagnoses. The International Disease Classification (ICD) Codes were used, together with the names of the different cardiac conditions. For the retrospective data collection there was total reliance on the compilation of the Medical Records Department for the period of study.

In terms of accuracy and reliability there are various inherent problems faced with these kinds of data. One obvious problem was the multiple dimensions of diseases suffered by in-patients in particular. In the present analysis each disease suffered by the patient has been recorded, since we were in no position to identify the major health problem. Hence some patients carried multiple recordings. In addition, it was not possible to identify the residential locations of some of the patients whose workplace addresses were used.

By and large, the data can be regarded as reliable. The diagnosis of cardiac diseases often goes through rigorous analysis by the physician and more often than not, a specialist (medical practitioner) makes the final diagnostic decision. With respect to the study area, Ibadan epitomises the sort of residential structure expected in most traditional-modern urban centres of Third World countries. In addition, the University of Ibadan Teaching Hospital (UCH) is one of the oldest and the best on the African continent, with an excellent medical records department. The Ring Road State Hospital is of comparative status while the Jericho Nursing Home is still staffed by excellent doctors who attend mainly to senior public servants in the State.

Data analysis and major findings

During the prospective study period (1989-90) there were about 854 in-patients suffering from cardiac diseases. Out of these, 102 cases were simply referred to as heart-related diseases. Of all the total number of cardiac cases, 66.5% were treated at UCH, 25.7% at the RRSH and only 7.8% at the JNH. The results of the data analysis indicated that more males were affected by cardiac disease and the fatality rates ranged between 24% and 26%.

Sex distribution of cardiac disease

As can be observed on Table 13.1, hypertensive heart disease topped the list of cardiac diseases, contribution 28% to the total number of cases. This was followed by peripheral vascular disease (17.8%), followed by myocarditis (12.9%), pulmonary heart disease (6.0%) and rheumatic heart disease (3.7%). To a large extent the present distribution

Table 13.1
Sex distribution of cardiac cases

Disease condition & ICD Code	Hospital									Total			
	UCH.			Ring Road State Hospital			Jericho Nursing Home						
	M	F	Total	M	F	Total	M	F	Total	M	F	Total	%
1. Rheumatic heart disease 391-398	11	21	32	-	-	-	1	-	1	12	21	33	3.9
2. Hypertensive heart disease 401-405	110	68	178	10	31	41	6	14	20	126	113	239	28.4
3. Ischaemic heart disease 410-414	7	7	14	-	-	-	-	-	-	7	7	14	1.7
4. Pulmonary heart disease 415-417	13	19	32	2	4	6	7	6	13	22	29	51	6.1
5. Other forms of heart disease	49	58	107	3	8	11	1	1	2	53	67	120	14.3
6. Cerebro-vascular disease 430-438	5	10	15	-	2	2	-	-	-	5	12	17	2.0
7. Peripheral vascular disease 440-448	37	38	75	17	50	67	8	2	10	62	90	152	18.1
8. Myocarditis 422	32	8	40	18	45	63	4	3	7	54	56	110	13.1
9. Cardiomyopathy 425	-	3	3	-	-	-	-	-	-	-	3	3	0.4
10. Other heart-related diseases	na	na	98	na	na	2	na	na	2	na	na	102	12.1
Total	264	232	594	50	140	192	27	26	55	341	398	841	
Per cent of total medical cases			44.25%			51.89%			16.5%			(37.08)	
11. Other medical conditions on admission na	na	752	na	na	370	na	na	327	na	na	697	na	

142

conforms with the results of some other previous studies. In particular, the present analysis still confirms the pre-eminence of hypertension among the commonest cardiac diseases in the urban centres of developing countries.

The sex distribution of the patients suffering from cardiac diseases was of some interest. For the purpose of this aspect of the analysis, it is preferable to concentrate more on the use of the more comprehensive data from the UCH and compare with the two other study hospitals. On the whole, more males suffer from hypertension, the leading cardiac disease in Ibadan city as well as many urban centres in developing countries. Likewise, more males appear to suffer from myocarditis.

On the other hand, more females consistently suffer from rheumatic heart disease, pulmonary heart disease and cerebrovascular disease as depicted in Table 13.1. The differentials observed at the RRSH and JNH may be due to incompleteness of the data of the two hospitals. It was only possible to collect complete data from the female medical wards at the RRSH, for instance.

Age composition of the cardiac patients

In any disease study, the distribution of the age-groups of the population at risk is usually of great concern. It is of interest to note that children carry the least risk of cardiac attack in the study area. As expected, individuals aged 45 and above bear the greatest risk of being afflicted with cardiac disease. Thus, on Table 13.2, about 64% of the patients were not less than 45 years old. It is also of significance to note that age-groups 25-34 years and 35-44 years appear now to carry equal risk of suffering from cardiac disease.

Table 13.2

Age distribution of cardiac cases

Age group	Number of cases	Percent
12 and under	2	0.3
12-24	64	9.8
25-34	82	12.5
35-44	91	13.9
45 and above	417	63.6
Total	656	100.0

Considering the relationship between age group and some specific cardiac diseases, it is noted that persons under age 24 years suffer mostly from rheumatic heart disease.

Seasonal distribution of cardiac admissions, 1989-1990

In the present analysis, there is really no undue emphasis on the relationship between seasonal variations and severity of cardiac attacks. Since climatic conditions are of least correlates in the literature. Nonetheless, it is gratifying to observe that most admissions occurred generally at the UCH and the city at large during the month of August followed by March, June, January, October and to some extent April. In August, most parts of southern Nigeria experience relatively low rains, hence August serves as a break between two marked rainy peaks. The weather phenomena are often unpredictable with little rain being followed by little sunshine. During the month of March the weather can be said to be 'nasty' as the heat bites, while rain expectation may be minimal, making conditions quite uncomfortable. Table 13.3 depicts the monthly distribution of cardiac cases. The seasonal pattern of the cause group may be of interest if only to know the type of relationship that exists between hospital and admissions of cardiac patients and the changes in the weather conditions.

Table 13.3

Monthly distribution of admission cases in study hospitals

Month	UCH		Ring Road State Hospital		Jericho		Total	
January	47	9.34	13	7.10	8	(15.38)	68	(9.21)
February	40	8.0	5	2.7	1	(1.9)	46	(6.2)
March	53	10.5	17	9.3	4	(7.7)	74	(10.0)
April	45	9.0	18	9.8	-	(0.0)	63	(8.5)
May	28	5.57	24	13.11	2	(3.85)	54	(7.3)
June	39	7.75	26	14.21	7	(13.46)	72	(9.7)
July	38	7.55	20	10.93	5	(9.62)	63	(8.5)
August	53	10.5	19	10.4	8	(15.4)	80	(10.8)
September	36	7.16	9	4.92	8	(15.38)	53	(7.2)
October	50	9.94	11	6.0	5	(9.6)	65	(8.8)
November	39	7.8	12	6.6	-	(0.0)	51	(6.9)
December	35	7.0	9	4.9	4	(8.0)	48	(6.5)
Total	503		183		52		738	998

Spatial distribution of cardiac patients during the study period, 1989-90

It is known in the literature that the incidence of cardiac diseases often coincide with changes in societal lifestyles. It has been alleged that socio-domestic environmental factors are of significance in the occurrence of cardiac diseases in any community.

Hence, it is of tremendous importance to identify the relative risks carried by different residential areas in any city and for the purpose of this analysis, in Ibadan metropolis. To achieve this objective, the city was roughly divided into three, namely, the core or inner city, the outer city and the periphery or suburbs of the city (Fig. 13.1). Table 13.4 indicates the spatial distribution of the admission cases within the study period by hospital.

Altogether, about 74% of all the admitted cardiac patients of the three study hospitals came within the city limits. In addition some 7% of others who came from the city used their workplace addresses. Also to emphasize the importance of the quality of the health care provided by the study hospitals for this kind of diseases, some 16% (and about 20% in UCH) of the patients came from other states of the country to receive treatment.

The distribution of the cardiac patients within the city is of great concern. In each of the three study hospitals that are located in different geographical areas (See Figure 13.1) of the city, the most modern section of the city, principally occupied by relatively wealthy individuals and senior civil servants, sent in majority of the admission cases. The core areas of the city carry a higher risk compared with the outer city. In each instance, the modern section of the city tends to carry not less than two-folds of its expected risk compared with the outer city. The implication of this distribution is that the relatively wealthy and by and large those who often occupy key social and economic positions in the society tend to bear the highest risks of cardiac attack.

People in the core area may be subject to stress related to poverty, while the desire to maintain a high social standing and secure a high lifestyle may have induced the high incidence of cardiac diseases in the suburbs. The corollary of these is that the people of the inner city are more contented or are resigned to their economic fate and thus suffer least from cardiac diseases.

The trend of cardiac morbidity in Ibadan city, 1957-1990

It is a known fact that increase in incidence of cardiac disease in any society is seen to be positively associated with levels of urbanization, industrialization and parameters of modernization in general. Hence, an analysis of the retrospective annual attendance and incidence rates data for a period of 34 years was done for UCH. Table 13.5 shows the distribution of the patients that attended the cardiac clinics at the hospital for the specified period and the incidence rates per 100,000 persons based on annual growth rate of 2.5% in spite of the inherent problems of the Nigerian population figures (other rates are also available for Ibadan City (Ayeni 6%, 1981 annual growth rate and Abumere 4.8% 1988 for Nigerian towns).

As can be observed on Table 13.5, the calculated incidence rates range from 82 in 1957 to 542 in 1978. Despite the inconsistency in the rates, the general impression shows much lower rates late in the 1950s and early 1960s. In contrast, the general rates are higher in the 1970s and 80s compared with 1950s and 1960s. On the whole, the highest rates are recorded in 1978 and 1982 followed by 1987, 1966, 1973-1976, 1965, 1988 and 1979 (See Table 13.5).

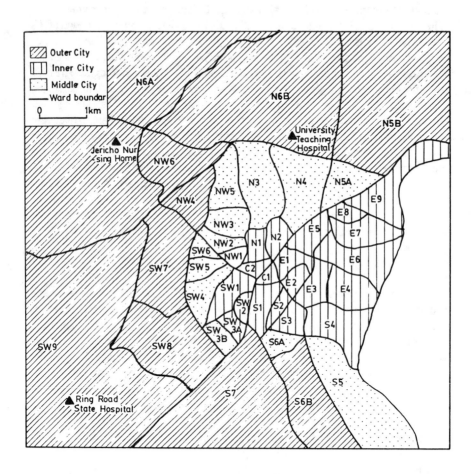

Figure 13.1 Residential structure of Ibadan city

Table 13.4
Spatial distribution of admission cases

Hospital	Residential areas							
	Ibadan				Other localities			All cases
	Inner city	Outer city	Suburb	City Total	Rest of Oyo state	Other states	Official addresses	
University College Hospital	127 (33.07)	89 (23.18)	168 (43.75)	384 (65.98)	12 (1.94)	123 (19.87)	33 (16.16)	552
Ring Road State Hospital	53 (32.32)	27 (16.46)	84 (51.22)	164 (28.18)	7 (3.83)	1 (0.55)	11 (6.01)	183
Jericho Nursing Home	3 (8.82)	2 (5.88)	29 (85.29)	34 (5.84)	1 (1.92)	3 (5.77)	14 (26.92)	52
Total	183 (31.44)	118 (20.27)	281 (48.28)	582 (73.95)	20 (2.54)	127 (16.14)	58 (7.37)	787

For further analysis, the cases treated were collated into five year intervals. The trend that emerges from this analysis has been displayed in Fig. 13.2. The figure, however confirms a consistent increase in the numbers attending the cardiac clinic at the University College Hospital in Ibadan. The implication of this trend is that the incidence of cardiac disease has increased with time since Nigeria's independence in 1960.

Discussion

Previous analyses of hospital-based records of cardiac diseases have shown the relative importance of this cause group to the overall admissions in African cities (Edington, 1954; D'Arbela, 1966; Carlisle and Ogunlesi, Akinkugbe, 1992 among others). Besides, evidence of increase in the incidence of cardiac disease in developing societies is becoming more apparent.

An earlier study by Edington (1954) in the then Gold Coast (present Ghana) confirmed that hypertension was not rare during the 1921-1953 study period. In spite of the smallness in the number of cases in the autopsies studied, more males than females died of hypertension. Even though D'Arbela (1966) reported that rheumatic heart disease often tops the list of cardiac diseases in Africa, followed directly by hypertension, the UCH data analyzed by him demonstrated the leading role of hypertension in Ibadan city. This distribution was further confirmed later by Carlisle and Ogunlesi (1972). Indeed, Carlisle and Ogunlesi confirmed the lead of hypertension in studies of other African cities such as Johannesburg, Cape Town, Kampala and Addis Ababa. Furthermore, in 1972, Falase corroborated the fact that Nigerians suffer more from hypertension compared with other cardiac conditions.

To a large extent, the results of the present study are in line with the previous studies that acclaimed the significance of hypertension. In 1991, hypertension still contributed some 28.0% (in perfect comparison with the 28% contribution discussed by Carlisle and Ogunlesi in 1972). There appears to be a slight decrease in the incidence of rheumatic heart disease. In this study it has contributed 3.7% as against 13.3% recorded by Carlisle and Ogunlesi in the 1972 UCH data.

What is more significant in the results of this study and the previous ones for UCH, is that more males were discovered to carry higher risk of cardiac diseases than females, especially in the incidence of hypertension. However, more females suffer from pulmonary heart disease and rheumatic heart disease. Less reliance is being placed on the data from Ring Road State Hospital and the Jericho Nursing Home as their facility definitively to diagnose cardiac cases is not as sophisticated as at the University College Hospital.

In the three study hospitals, the case fatality rate was about 25.5%, which is relatively high. Besides, cardiac admissions contributed 44.3 to 51.9% of all medical admissions in the two specialist hospitals (UCH and RRSH).

Table 13.5
Yearly clinic attendance and incidence rates of cardiac cases at the UCH, 1957-90

Year	Estimated population	Total attendance	Rate per 100,000	Year	Estimated polulation	Total attendance	Rate per 100,000
1958	552,781	905	164	1975	843,754	3,310	392
1959	566,955	1,409	247	1976	864,848	3,543	410
1960	581,492	1,555	267	1977	886,469	3,582	404
1961	596,402	1,356	277	1978	908,631	4,925	542
1962	611,694	1,546	253	1979	931,346	3,665	393
1963	627,379	1,391	222	1980	954,630	3,449	361
1964	643,063	2,177	339	1981	978,496	4,228	432
1965	659,136	2,624	398	1982	1,002,958	5,419	540
1966	675,618	2,751	407	1983	1,028,032	3,337	325
1967	692,508	1,990	287	1984	1,053,733	3,387	321
1968	709,821	2,603	367	1985	1,080,076	3,239	300
1969	727,567	2,814	387	1986	1,107,078	3,955	357
1970	745,756	2,539	340	1987	1,134,755	5,075	446
1971	764,400	2,402	314	1988	1,163,124	4,604	396
1972	783,500	2,807	358	1989	1,192,202	3,935	330
1973	803,098	3,538	440	1990	1,220,007	3,919	321

The spatial dimension of the cardiac admissions was of tremendous interest in this study. The most modern section of the city, which is often occupied by enlightened and well to do individuals, carries the highest risk of cardiac disease. This aspect of the results requires some emphasis. To begin with, increase in the incidence of cardiac diseases has often been closely associated with changes in lifestyles of individuals. In particular a change from conservative traditional lifestyle into modern and sophisticated lifestyles as they affect consumption patterns and acquisition of modern habits such as cigarette smoking, alcohol consumption often elevate the incidence of cardiac disease.

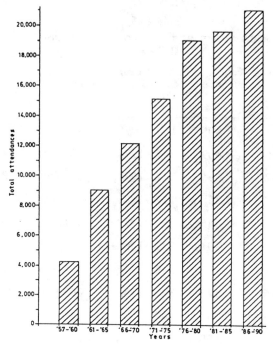

Figure 13.2   Trend of five year total attendance of cardiac patients at the University College Hospital (UCH) GOP department, 1957-1990.

The suggestion is that as our society moves from traditional living conditions to modern or sophisticated living standards, which often implies advance in national development, there is the tendency of the affluent to carry higher risks of cardiac diseases. Besides this, the fact that the most modern areas of Ibadan city reported more cases of cardiac diseases during the study period, one other aspect of the spatial pattern of the diseases was of interest. In each of the three study hospitals, the core area of the city was well represented. This suggests that this relatively poor segment of the city is afflicted by poverty related stress conditions which predispose the people to cardiac diseases. This suggestion also goes a long way to confirm the close relationship between cardiac morbidity and national development. In this study, it has been confirmed as expected that males suffer more than females, especially in the incidence of hypertension. In general, men are more mobile and aggressive in the pursuit of modern lifestyles and often react more poorly to economic shocks than females. It is therefore not surprising to discover that males carry higher risks than females.

What is also of concern is the age distribution of the population at greatest risk. The ages that are most prone to cardiac morbidity are those above 45 years. This is the period when most individuals and in particular men are most aggressive in their socio-economic pursuits. It will not be surprising if indeed a lot of deaths explained by "unnatural" or "undetermined" factors in our societies are accounted for by cardiac attacks. It is therefore necessary to carry out more of this type of study and educate our population, especially those who have reached the age of 45 years, about the need for regular medical examinations.

Conclusion

In conclusion, national development which infers changes in the lifestyles of individuals is concomitant with the tendency for wealthy individuals to be susceptible to cardiac disease.

The age composition of the cardiac in-patients indicates the tendency for individuals aged 45 and above to bear the greatest risks. In addition, those who occupy the most modern section of the city are mostly affected while those in the core area carry the next relatively high risk.

The importance of the study should be of national concern to our health planners. It appears the Nigerian society is in the epidemiological transition and the increase in the cardiac morbidity requires urgent analysis. First, besides the relatively high case fatality associated with such a morbidity cause group it is expensive to treat such patients. It is therefore important to incorporate regular medical examinations in our primary health care. Secondly, health education is required for both the most affluent and the medium affluent members of the society as well as the skilled professionals to prevent their avoidable death. Rapid redevelopment of the core area and the provision of basic facilities in particular, is called for to reduce possible environmentally-promoted stress conditions.

References

Carlisle, R. and Ogunlesi, T.O. (1972), 'Prospective study of adult cases presenting at the Cardiac Unit, UCH, Ibadan 1968 and 1969'. *Afr. J. Med. Sci.* 3, 13-25.

D'Arbela, P.G., Kanyerezi, R.B. and Tulloch, J.A. (1966), 'A study of heart disease in the Mulago Hospital, Kampala, Uganda'. *Trans. Roy. Soc. Trop Med., Hyg.*, 60, 782-790.

Edington, G.M. (1954), 'Cardiovascular disease as a cause of death in the Ghanian'. *Trans Roy. Soc. Trop Med. Hyg.* 48, 419.

Falase, A.O. and Osuntokun, B.O. (1972), Myocardial infraction in Nigerians. *Trop. Geog. Med.*, 25, 147-150.

Hellen, J.A. (1978), 'Geomedicine and the quality of life: patterns of mortality and morbidity under conditions of rapid change': Seminar paper, United Nations Cairo Demographic Centre.

Hellen, J.A. (1982), 'Western Diseases: Their Emergence and Prevention'. *Science and Public Policy* 9, 4:269-73.

14 Tourist health and tourist medicine in the tropics: A case for sustainable development?

J. Anthony Hellen

Summary

The main theme of the chapter is the critical importance of medical geographical/geomedical research in the planning and development of a sustainable tourist sector in developing countries. It outlines the historic development of tropical medicine and traces the growth of the global tourist industry to its collective position as the world's largest business.

The marked expansion of both medical and non-medical literature relating directly and indirectly to the health risks of international travel, and to the wider issues of tourist management and public health, is reviewed before the question of imported tropical disease and pre-travel advice is illustrated by reference to British experience. Finally, the globalization of leisure is linked with the scope for medical-geographical research in areas like disease hazard mapping and the dynamics of disease ecology, given the growing demand for high quality health information from an industry concerned by consumer legislation and the risks of medical litigation by its customers.

Introduction

With the rapid increase of international travel and tourism, tourist health and tourist medicine are attracting growing attention in both the medical literature and the medical profession. It will be argued that parallel to this situation, geography and particularly medical geography have potentially important contributions to make in areas of applied research and consultancy within government planning agencies in developing countries and in the private sector tourist industry more generally. Mass tourism is expected to become the world's biggest industry by the year 2000, and the implications of this make agreement on a comprehensive research agenda an urgent priority.

Mention of sustainability in the title is deliberately ambiguous. As a key component of development in many developing countries, tourism is highly vulnerable to internal and external shocks as varied as recession, international conflicts, natural disasters and epidemic disease. Sustainable tourism therefore requires a deep understanding not only of economics and international relations, but also of the geoecology which underpins and ultimately constrains much actual and potential tropical and sub-tropical tourism. In an article on Belize, Pearce has highlighted this problem in noting that preparation of development plans for tourism has been "largely the responsibility of professional planners, economists, marketing consultants, and architects"; the input from geographers he describes as meagre (Pearce, 1984). Like many branches of manufacturing industry today tourism, as a service industry, seems nevertheless likely to be driven by a combination of legislation and commercial self-interest, consumer demand shareholder pressure to incorporate *environmental impact assessment* and *environmental audit* as routine management and planning tools. The epidemiological and public health ramifications of transient tourist populations exposed to unprecedented disease hazards will in addition necessitate the widespread use of *environmental risk assessment* as well. Sustainable tourism in the developing countries will require a maintenance programme of disease prevention and geomedical surveillance in the sending and receiving areas, which the medical profession alone is quite incapable of delivering.

This paper therefore takes as its starting point the historical dimension of travellers' health and disease in the tropics, with particular reference to the growth and decline of the European schools of tropical medicine and the inexorable rise of popular tourism. That there are obvious links between exploration, colonialism, the Golden Age of microbiology, and the classic infections is clear, and it is not without its irony that the president of the World Travel and Tourism Council was reported in 1992 as describing tourism as a "new form of colonialism" acting as a *parasite* (my italics) on the emaciated Third World (*The Times*, 17 November 1992).

The dictionary definition of parasitism as an intimate association between organisms of different kinds, involving a dependence on something else for existence or support, is a useful conceptual link between apparently unconnected aspects of the benefits and risks of this global industry. It serves to underline the dangers of conducting research into tourism in the developing world without recalling how, little over a century ago, indigenous tropical diseases had baffled a medical world whose knowledge was restricted to illnesses of temperate areas (cf. Ransford, 1983; Hellen, 1986), but it also opens up the prospect that global tourism may itself become a vehicle for investment in environmental health programmes and securing improved health for all.

The growth of international travel and the structural changes within the international tourist industry area of relevance here, from the aspect of tourism management and of public health responses. These latter range from the global responsibilities of the World Health Organisation to the advisory role of national governments and the industry's representative in providing travellers with information on protecting their health and avoiding hazards. Any reading of the literature within geography will confirm the increased interest in links between tourism resources and national development planning in tropical countries as varied as Indonesia (Hussey, 1989), India (Bender, 1993) Rwanda (Gotanegre, 1992) and Thailand (Peyrou, 1992), but the question of health hazards and imported disease generally occupies - if any - a place behind research into the environmental impacts of tourism, socio-economic change and economic restructuring, or growing concern for safeguarding the environment and preserving societies and cultures under the aegis of a new "eco-tourism".

In this review recent research and routinely collected epidemiological data on Britain are used to establish the scale of imported infections. One research area deserving closer attention is the promotion and marketing of exotic holiday destinations, whether within mass charter tourism or the specialized adventure and wilderness companies in travel brochures. The sheer scale of this "literature" is evident in the fact that the British travel industry alone prints 120 million holiday brochures a year costing £86.5 million, at a cost of £20 for each booking (Green Flag International, 1993).

Their contents and information sources deserve much closer study than heretofore and, in the face of such saturation of the market, raise questions of the travel industry's "duty to care" for its customers and of the medical profession's legal liabilities and self-interest in underlining the growing need for provision of pre- and post-travel health advice to all such travellers, based on both medical and geomedical information.

Parallel to developments reported on or implicit in the "grey" literature of the travel companies, and in that of the medical profession, there has been a significant recent growth of specialized journals dealing with health, disease and travel, as well as in the convening of conferences and courses responding to these issues and unmet needs. This paper reviews some of these opportuned responses in terms of their wider importance in defining and redefining the future tasks of an applied medical geography operating at the interface with a world industry and a global phenomenon shaped by commercial enterprise and consumer responses.

Finally, the subject is related to the tasks which medical geographers might undertake in the future, by "recycling" existing materials and knowledge, and adapting methods and approaches used outside the tropics and sub-tropics, and by undertaking research into disease hazard mapping and the dynamics of disease ecology. It is suggested that these could form an essential contribution to and component of the planning and operation of a *sustainable* tourist industry, whether in the sending or the receiving countries. The wisdom of running down the schools of tropical medicine with the ending of colonial empires could be questioned, and the urgency of revising Western medical training and undergraduate curricula to accommodate changing circumstances and the globalization of leisure is at least arguable.

Tropical medicine

Traditionally the great tomes of tropical medicine (cf. Adams and Maegraith, 1989) have presented an encyclopedic account of the major infections and parasitic maladies of the "tropics", often loosely described as "the hot, developing countries of low latitudes". Although great attention has necessarily been paid to the clinical picture, most such textbooks devote considerable and commendable space to detail such as the ecology and life cycles of parasites, intermediate hosts and vectors, and to outlining the "geographical distribution" and aetiology and defining endemicity. Indeed, in the last revision of their *Clinical Tropical Diseases* (op. cit. above, p.iv) the authors noted that:

> "the export/import of disease...today affects every doctor who examines a patient, wherever he may be. In the routine interrogation of every patient, the doctor, or nurse, or whoever sees him first, must *automatically obtain the geographical history* (their italics). The major element in spreading diseases across the world has been the aeroplane".

Similarly, in the second edition of *Tropical and Geographical Medicine*, the introductory contributor, D A Warrell, reiterates the increasing significance of imported tropical diseases, noting that:

> "No doctor can now afford to ignore the increasing problem of imported tropical disease created by the boom in travel to tropical areas...it is very useful to have an atlas in the travel clinic so that the itinerary can be understood" (Warren and Mahmoud, 1990, p.2).

Tropical medicine is unique in being a "vertical speciality" defined by the part of the world in which the illness is acquired. Its development from the preceding military schools of medicine to the schools of tropical medicine in Europe from the close of the 19th century (the first School of Tropical Medicine was founded at Liverpool in 1889) is perhaps too well known to detail here, but the growth of centres like those in London, Liverpool, Antwerp, Hamburg and Marseilles during the colonial era was in time matched by that of research institutes in the tropical continents themselves. Eventually tropical medicine was transformed to a "medicine in the tropics" and ultimately to a concern with the diseases of poverty and global communicable diseases. It is no small irony that this renewed interest in the old tropical pathogens is linked with the "new" or exotic diseases of affluence and global travel, and it invests the earlier work of such medical pioneers such as Manson, Ross, and Castellani with new importance.

It might be argued that, apart from conceptual confusion over the place of tropical medicine in contemporary medicine, much expertise based on fieldwork in the tropics has been sacrificed with the advance of more "modern" medicine, and that the subject is due for a major re-activation under rapidly changing relations between the tropics and non-tropics. The "tropicalization" of areas in the sub-tropics as a consequence of global warming has enormous public health implications for the tourism industry as disease vectors or alien species extend their range (cf. Godlee, 1991; Burgos et al 1991; Hansen and Fung, 1988). At least two areas of concern suggest themselves: the first lies in the field of medical training and the health advisory role of general practitioners, and is outside the present discussion; the second lies in the field of the agencies involved in inadvertently promoting the risk-taking activity of longhaul, but generally short-stay, tourist migration.

Where an earlier age was concerned with exploration by Europeans and the health and disease dimension of travel and employment in tropical areas reflected in, for example, the many editions of the Royal Geographical Society's *Hints to Travellers (RGS 1854-1938)* or the publisher, John Murray's *Guides and Handbooks from 1835, today the modern tourist industry has resurrected or coined phrases like explorer, elite and off-beat* in an attempt to segment and add value to a market dominated by the charter and mass tourism sectors, but arguably without giving sufficient thought to pre-travel advice and information through its (travel) agents to reflect these lifestyle changes (cf. Cossar et al. 1993). A growing minority of travellers is prepared to pay (often highly) for adventurous and sometimes physically or pathogenically risky holidays, attracted by such descriptions as "low-impact wilderness living" or trekking in "the world's most beautiful and remote regions", but without realizing that the health information provided may induce a false sense of security.

Wide reading in the medical literature will demonstrate a growing concern in the profession for health risks, whether those affecting particular destinations and countries or travellers' behaviour. Profiles of *travellers at risk* (Table 14.1) and of the *high risk areas* themselves (Figure 14.1) are likely in future to be progressively refined at the behest of the insurance industry, and the scope for such environmental advice and consultancy by medical geographers is therefore already considerable.

Table 14.1
Profile of travellers at risk

Package holiday makers	>other travellers
Inexperienced travellers	>other travellers
Travellers further south, particularly Northern Africa	>other travellers
Summer travellers	>winter travellers
Younger age groups (specially 20-29 years)	>older age groups
Smokers	>non-smokers

Source: WHO, 1989

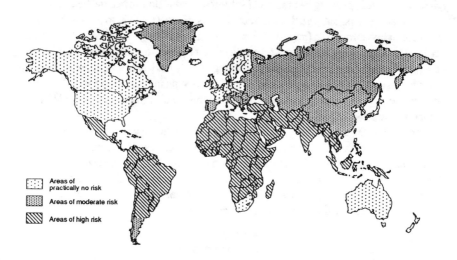

Figure 14.1   Global health risk areas

(Source: Le Soir, 23/24 May 1992, after Steffen and L'Association Medasso)

Tourism studies and the growth of tourism

The non-medical literature

If the quantity of published literature is any guide, tourism represents an area of sustainable growth for academic writers and publishers alike, although much of it runs parallel to the ephemeral trade journalism. Tourism Abstracts cover most of the major tourism periodicals, whilst research literature is already concentrated in journal like the *Annals of Tourism Research, the Journal of Travel-Research and Tourism Management.* Others like *Travel and Tourism Analyst, Tourist Review, Tourism Intelligence Quarterly* and the *WTO's Travel Research Journal* are of value, and the Economist Intelligence Unit's quarterly *Travel and Tourism Analyst* provides highly focused reports. Geographical journals as different has *Environment and Planning* (cf. Britton, 1991) and the Cahiers d'Outre-Mer (cf. Salomon, 1992) have published an increasing range of papers relevant to the topic under discussion.

The World Tourism Organization, a United Nations body, produces a range of statistics on the industry, particularly the *Yearbook of Tourism Statistics* and the *Tourism Compendium*, as well as the *Travel Research Journal*. Although wide in their coverage, textbooks within the general field of tourism are clearly targeted in the main to a readership with specific training or information needs. Some, like *The Tourist Business* (Lundberg, 1990) are unusual in dealing with health and travel, and the same author's *International Travel and Tourism* (Lundberg and Lundberg, 1988) includes health and the prevalence of disease in a ranking of the "top ten" and the "dirty dozen" countries (to be avoided by tourists), with Switzerland heading the former and Chad occupying the bottom place in the latter.

The tourism industry

It is sometimes forgotten that one of the most important motives in 18th century Britain for travel to mainland Europe was to combine tourism and travelling for health; continental watering places like Spa and Aachen established a fashion (Black, 1992). But parallels with today are to be found two centuries and more ago, before the "Grand Tour" declined into the "package tour", when ill health whilst travelling was already recognised as a serious problem. Although diseases like malaria were feared in parts of Italy, and there were echoes of contemporary concerns over sexually transmitted diseases (the 1739 *Gentleman's Guide* alerted readers to the risk of contracting veneral diseases in southern France), "much of the ill health suffered was intestinal, due to bad water and poorly-prepared food", and a "large number of British travellers died abroad" (Black, 1992, pp. 188-89 and 1991).

The modern growth of popular tourism from Europe is associated, along with the American Express Company, with the name of Thomas Cook, who organized his first excursions in the 1840s and who filled trains and steamships by setting up ticket agencies and accessory services, thereby creating tourism in the contemporary sense (Pemble, 1991; Brendon, 1991) - in the words of a mid-nineteenth century critic, "reducing the traveller to the level of his trunk". As the literary historian Paul Fussell so memorably pointed out: "before tourism there was travel and before travel there was exploration. Each is roughly assignable to its own age in modern history: exploration belongs to the Renaissance, travel to the bourgeois age, tourism to our proletarian movement" (Fussell, 1989, p.38).

These phases have now been superseded by an age of mass tourism and multinational enterprise best summarized in Figure 14.2, demonstrating the inexorable rise in tourist numbers between 1960 and 1992, and in Table 14.2 which shows the numbers and market shares in today's global industry in the period 1985-1990. Europe still commands a roughly two-thirds share of the world total of 476 million tourists in 1992, and 640 million predicted by the WTO by the year 2000. South Asia had a mere 0.8% of this total and Africa a modest 3.3%, yet detailed figures for Africa in 1990, however, show total tourist arrivals of 17.7 million - a not inconsiderable number by contrast with 1960 when the one million mark was first reached, and substantially more than the Caribbean (11.4 million in 1990), but less than South East Asia (21.54 million in 1990), for example.

Global tourism has almost unnoticed become the world's largest business, travel alone generating in excess of US $2000 billion a year. Just as Thomas Cook's use of rail and water transport from 1841 transformed an industry, so the introduction of reliable jet aircraft in 1957 and of jumbo jets in 1970 revolutionized tourist movements and potential disease spread. It is estimated that between two-thirds and three-quarters of all travel by volume is now accounted for by tourism, and around 12% of the world economy is generated by it; 80% of all international travel is made by nationals from 20 countries, five of which account for over 50% of all travel expenditure (*The Economist*, 1991).

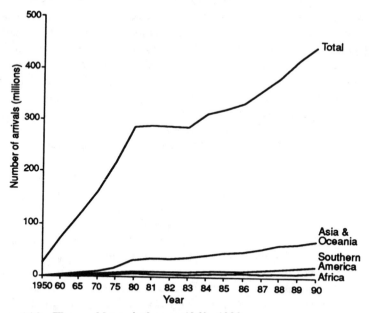

Figure 14.2   The world tourist boom: 1960 - 1992

Source: World Tourism Organization (WTO)

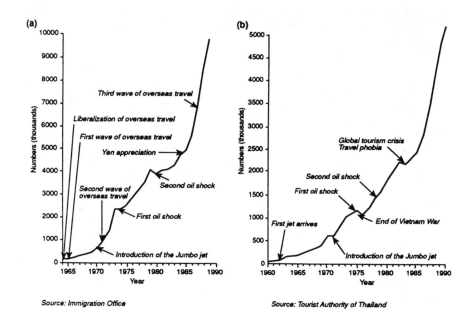

Figure 14.3   Sending and receiving: the development of mass tourist movements in Japan (a) and Thailand (b)

Case studies: Japan and Thailand

The growth of the Japanese tourist industry provides a particularly graphic case study of what may soon be repeated elsewhere in the Pacific Rim states, and its performance is compared with that of Thailand in Figure 14.3. Only in 1964 was overseas travel liberalized in Japan, and the first wave of tourist movements dates from 1965 when 369,000 tourists came to Japan and only 159,000 Japanese went overseas on holiday. By

1971 the outward movement for the first time exceeded one million travellers as the jumbo jet transformed the scale of operations. The oil shocks of 1973/74 and 1978 saw a temporary hiatus, but the appreciation of the Japanese yen underpinned a third wave of overseas travel which, by 1992, was expected to have passed the 11 million mark (Reiko, 1991).

The Japanese tourist industry is marked, moreover, by government sponsored "tourism infrastructure projects" worldwide, which include resorts in many tropical areas, including Thailand, Burma, Indonesia and the Philippines designed specifically for the Japanese clientele (Misato, 1991).

The case of Thailand, a mainly receiving country which had 635,555 Japanese visitors in 1990, provides similar evidence of the speed and scale of change.

The subject of tourism in Thailand is well documented (Peyrou, 1992; Hohnholz, 1984; King and Barnwell, 1992; Richter, 1989). Since the late-1950s Bangkok airport had become the main air transport node between South East Asia and Europe, Japan and Australasia (the first jet aircraft arrived in 1962), and since then the country has exemplified laisser-faire development and a tourist boom. The American involvement in the Vietnam war until 1975 led to the use of Thailand by its service personnel (maximally 543,000 in 1969) for "rest and recreation" and arguably laid the foundation of modern "sex tourism" in that country.

From a near standing-start in 1959, Thailand had passed the one million mark by 1973, 2 million by 1981, and 5 million by 1989. The 1990 total reached 5.29 million arrivals, with Western Europe providing 644,115 of these (Germany: 239,915; France: 194,618), slightly more than Japan's 635,000, and well ahead of the United States with 291,635 and Australia with 226, 785 tourist arrivals. Neighbouring Malaysia provided 804,629 arrivals and Singapore 289,411, however, Thailand's tropical location (6° 2^oN) and monsoon climate go some way to explain the relatively high risk of contracting tropical diseases, ranging from the insect-borne malaria and filariasis and dengue haemorrhagic fever, but the sexually transmitted diseases in have attracted most international interest. Although over 20 pathogens are involved in this STD group, HIV/AIDS have commanded most attention, and it is said that today's tourists assume the role formerly played by armies in spreading STDs (De Schryver and Meheus, 1989). "Holiday romance syndrome" aptly describes the heightened behavioural risks of contracting STDs on holiday; Porter et al. (1992) have estimated that an individual is 300 times more likely to contract HIV abroad than in Britain.

The Thailand case is particularly interesting, given that the first AIDS case there was diagnosed in late 1984, and until early 1988 there was complacency over the risk (Bernard, 1991), with only 7 cases of AIDS and 171 cases of HIV seropositives known to the HIV/AIDS Registry, most of whom were associated with intravenous (heroin) drug abuse. Even in mid-1989, the date of the "AIDS take-off" in both Japan and Thailand, the latter was reporting an AIDS incidence of 0.204 per 100,000 population, little more than Japan's

Table 14.2

International travel: arrivals by regions 1985–1990

	1985	1986	1987	1988	1989	1990	Av. annual growth	Market 1985	share 1990
	'000	'000	'000	'000	'000	'000	1985-1990	%	%
Europe	214,300	215,400	230,800	239,300	266,900	275,500	5.2	66.4	64.2
Americas	58,700	62,900	68,000	75,000	78,500	84,000	7.4	18.2	19.6
East Asia and Pacific	29,400	33,100	38,400	44,700	44,400	46,500	9.6	9.1	10.8
South Asia	2,500	2700	2,700	2,900	3,100	3,250	5.4	0.8	0.8
Middle East	8,000	6,900	7,000	7,400	7,800	6,000	-5.6	2.5	1.4
Africa	9800	9,500	10,000	12,600	13,600	14,000	7.4	3.0	3.3
World Total	322,700	330,500	356,800	381,900	414,200	429,250	5.9	100.0	100.0

Source: WTO, 1991

Table 14.3
Main infection risks in developing countries

Group	Risk		Disease
HIGH	>1case per 10 travellers	(2)	Diarrhoea Upper respiratory infection
MEDIUM	>1 case per 200, but <1 per 10 travellers		Dengue Enteroviral infection Food poisoning Gastroenteritis Giardiasis Hepatitis A
		(13)	malaria without prophylaxis Salmonellosis STDs Gonorrhoea Chlamydia infection Herpes simplex Nonspecific urethritis Shigellosis
LOW	>1 per 1000, but <1 per 200 travellers		Acute haemorrhagic conjunctivitis Amoebiasis Ascariasis Childhood infections Chickenpox Measles Mumps Poliomyelitis Enterobiasis
		(19)	Hepatitis B Hepatitis, non-A non-B (epidemic) Leptospirosis Scabies STDs Syphilis Chancroid Strongyloidiasis Trichuriasis Tropical sprue Tuberculosis Typhoid fever

Source: Warren and Mahmoud, 1990, Tropical & Geographical Medicine

0.113 (cf. USA - 14.15; Australia - 3.17; Germany - 1.83). With an estimated 500,000 - 700,000 prostitutes in the country, and a Thai culture which sanctions recourse to brothels, the mid-1993 estimate that there are now 600,000 HIV-infected Thais (1% of the total population) is a warning of impending catastrophe for the tourist industry, as for the country at large (Zeitung, 1993). By the year 2000 an estimated 2 million (or 3%) of the population will carry the infection and every third death will be from AIDS, at a cost to the country of at least US $2 billion per year in care and treatment - a figure higher than present annual foreign investment in the kingdom.

Health risks

In future studies of global disease patterns, it seems highly likely that medical historians and others will come to regard the global leisure revolution, exemplified by Japanese and Thai experience over the past two decades, coupled with global warming and climate change, as having contributed significantly to the broadening of the range of infections to which human beings had been exposed. Unprecedented contemporary changes in transport media and the movement of people between different climatic zones seems likely to have effects on global health and disease patterns as profound as many of those in history, which linked disease pools (cf. McNeill, 1977; Cohen, 1989; Howe, 1982

Growing concern for the health risks of international travel is consequently evident on many fronts. Tables 14.3 and 14.4 respectively act as an *aide-memoire* for the main (general) infection risks in developing countries, and highlight the long to very long incubation periods for certain largely tropical diseases.

In Table 14.3 the risk of infection may be higher than 1 in 10 travellers overall, and 13 well-known diseases are grouped under a medium risk of 1 case in 200, down to 1 in 10. Table 14.4 highlights 25 further infections which may incubate over periods from 1 to many years, by which time multiple holidays may have been enjoyed in a variety of risk areas. A further 22, not listed here but including dengue, gonorrhoea, relapsing fever and yellow fever take only one week or less to incubate and are in diagnostic terms a simpler problem than the iceberg of "delayed" infection likely to be hidden in some returnees.

A recent survey in Britain by the Consumers' Association analyzed responses from 3,713 holiday makers. Nearly 16% had reportedly suffered some form of illness on holiday. In terms of countries, 60% of those holidaying in Egypt, 47% in The Gambia, and 45% in both Turkey and Latin America reported illness (*Holiday Which* May 1991, p. 130). The most common complaints were stomach upsets, excess heat, travel sickness, and altitude sickness, rather than the infections listed earlier.

Other research reports highlight the numbers affected by travel to developing countries, including infections like malaria and AIDS, typhoid and hepatitis-B, as well as skin cancers (melanoma). One medical practitioner (Petty, 1989) makes the good point that "facing disease is never easy, but it must be anathema for an industry devoted to the promotion of pleasure". Nonetheless, the tourist is often literally the innocent abroad and the profession is increasingly facing up to the likelihood of medical negligence claims where vaccination and prophylaxis recommendations are ignored by patients (cf. J.D. Holden, 1989).

Table 14.4
Long to very long incubation periods

Long (1 to 6 months)	Very long (2 months to years)
Ascariasis	AIDS
Blastomycosis	Cysticercosis
Hepatitis B	Echinococcosis
Hepatitis delta	Filariasis
Hepatitis, non-A non-B	Fluke infection
(posttransfusion)	Leishmaniasis, visceral
Leishmaniasis, cutaneous	Leprosy
Loiasis	Schistosomiasis
Malaria	Trypanosomiasis, African
Melioidosis	(Gambian)
Pinta	
Rabies	
Taeniasis	
Trichuriasis	
Tropical sprue	
Yaws	

Source: Warren and Mahmoud, 1990

Responses from within medicine

I: Academic

The special issue of the *World Health Statistics Quarterly* (42, 1989) which dealt, inter alia, with health hazards of international travel, tourist health as a new branch of public health, sexually transmitted diseases, and malaria, marks something of a milestone in the present discussion, although Velimirovic, a senior WHO officer, had five years earlier discussed at some length the development of world tourism and the problem of imported tropical diseases in Europe, noting that "*the big influx of tropical diseases expected after the 1950s, when the large-scale increase in travel started, did not materialize except for malaria*" (Velimirovic, 1984: chapter 4; my italics).

The setting up of an Italian Association for Tourist Medicine at Rimini in 1983 led directly to the designation in 1988 of a WHO collaborating centre for tourist health and tourist medicine, with the aim ultimately of establishing an *International Association for Tourist Health*.

A number of medical journals outside the obvious sources like the *Reviews of Infectious Diseases*, or the *Transactions of the Royal Society of Tropical Medicine and Hygiene*, offer material of great potential interest to medical geographers in this border area with tourism and travel. One such is *Travel Medicine International*, which first appeared in 1983 as *Travel and Traffic Medicine International*, and is now subtitled the *Journal of Emporiatics* - from the Greek word *emporos* or traveller or trader - but the research literature appears to be growing exponentially, and it is not appropriate to attempt an overview here, except to note with interest the appearance of a new *Journal of Wilderness Medicine* in 1990, and the increasing numbers of travel medicine articles in leading journals like *The Lancet*, the *British Medical Journal*, the *Journal of the American Medical Association*, and the *New England Journal of Medicine*.

Several specialized symposia have occupied the international stage in recent years, and reflect the growing concern for these issues. The first *International Conference on Travel Medicine* was held in Zurich in April, 1988. One on *Travel and Tropical Medicine for South East Asia* was held in Bangkok in February, 1992, and targeted business people as well as the health sector. 1993 saw the *World Congress* on Tourist Medicine and Health in Singapore, and the International Travel Medicine conference in Paris. Other more specialized symposia have concentrated on particular risk environments - as in the one on *Infections and the Alpine Environment* held in Cortina, Italy in 1992, but it has to be noted that much medical writing continues only to cite literature from within its own discipline and to ignore the work of social and environmental scientists.

In this context mention should be made of timely global review conducted by the American Institute of Medicine, which has reported on emerging microbial *threats* to human health in the United States from old and new infections, and the *factors* (ranging from microbial adaptation and land use to human behaviour) shaping the *process of emergence* (Lederberg et al, 1992).

With appendices providing a comprehensive 60-page catalogue of infectious disease agents, and ranging from arboviruses such as the hantavirus group (HFRS etc) and the filoviruses (Ebola, Lassa etc), to HIV I and II and resurgent TB and malaria, the report is of wide international significance, and follows a linked report on *The US. Capacity to Address Tropical Infectious Disease Problems* (IOM 1987). Yet despite the collaboration of a 19-member inter-disciplinary committee representing 15 subject areas, only 4 sides of its substantive text of 169 pages are devoted to international travel as a factor in emergence, no geographer was reportedly involved in the working parties, and the bibliography lacks all reference to research from within medical geography or geomedicine in the United States or abroad and almost totally ignores foreign language literature.

Imported tropical disease and pre-travel health advice: the British case

The British travel industry is well established, with most overseas travel booked through travel agents and tourist movements being well documented. Although overshadowed by Germany, the world's leading origin market in terms of foreign tourism, with 69 million trips abroad in 1991, United Kingdom residents made 33.4 million visits abroad in 1992 and a record 18.1 overseas visitors arrived (BTA/ETB, 1993). The period 1949 - 1991 saw a 53-fold increase in the numbers travelling beyond Europe (Cossar et al, 1993), and this was accompanied by a notable rise in imported infections.

Data on notifiable and some other diseases imported into the British Isles are relatively easily obtained from the Public Health Laboratory Services in London and the Communicable Diseases (Scotland) Unit (CDSU) in Glasgow. Although most travellers' illnesses

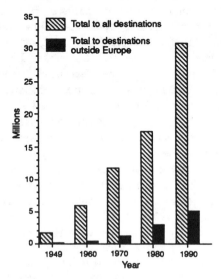

Source: J Cossar et al 1993

Figure 14.4   Visits abroad by United Kingdom residents: 1949 - 1990

go unreported, the general level of health problems has been widely investigated (cf. Layton and Bia, 1992 for a valuable bibliography). Steffen el al. (1987) estimated that about 15% of Americans returning from developing countries experienced health problems, with 8% consulting a physician; a survey over the period 1973-1985 suggested a 37% level of travel-related illness (Cossar et al, 1990). Cossar et al list 24 infections imported into the U.K in the period 1978-1988, ranging from AIDS (HIV), amoebiasis, brucellosis, giardiasis, leishmaniasis, leptospirosis, rabies, schistosomiasis and trypanosomiasis to the classic immunizable infections like cholera, hepatitis (A & B) and typhoid/paratyphoid.

The growth in numbers of imported malaria infections is well documented and accords with its widespread distribution in the tropics and subtropics, the well-publicized concern for reported chloroquine and mefloquine resistance by *Plasmodium falciparum* and *P. vivax*, and increasing travel to endemic areas (cf. Phillips-Howard et al 1988; Wyler, 1983). More than 8000 Europeans a year reportedly contract malaria, and by 1991 2,300 imported cases resulted in 13 deaths in Britain; Figure 14.5 graphs the numbers of imported cases from the three tropical continents for the period 1981-1990, and the regional breakdown for Africa. The decline in cases originating in Asia from a 1986 peak contrasts starkly with a rise in African numbers from 400 to nearly 1100 by 1990. The high risk status of West Africa, with 228 cases in 1981 and 675 cases in 1990 is evident, but the increase in the main Africa tourist region of East Africa is a particular threat to the tourist industry, given recent negative publicity in the British media.

The European newspaper (23 July, 1992) carried a detailed article under the headline "Tourists die as malaria defies drugs", and *The Times* (13 May, 1993) printed a headline "Britons warned as malaria spreads" over an article about the death of a tourist. (Significantly, the director of the Kenya National Tourist Office in London wrote to *The European* a week later that the African Medical and Research Foundation, based in Nairobi, had issued a statement that: "The risk of malaria in East Africa is less than in West Africa and the situation has improved over the last few years. In fact, prompt and proper treatment of malaria should always be successful").

Nonetheless, alongside six coloured maps of "World diseases: areas of risk" - which included malaria in Kenya - *The Times* (23 August, 1993) headlined a global warning by the WHO urging tourists to take seriously the hazards of disease abroad with the words "Britons on holiday face growing risk of disease". It would be difficult to imagine a more negative form of publicity for an industry predicated on carefree enjoyment.

Health advice

Although medical geography has no direct part to play in health advice to travellers, the geomedical monitoring and surveillance of changing disease distributions and health hazards needs to be fed back into the information systems on which preventative medical advice is based. Ideally, medical students should, in a world of what Epstein (1993) has called "global village viruses", routinely receive instruction in medical geography/geomedicine,as they do in epidemiology, business management, and psychology. Maegraith's question "*Unde Venis?*" (From whence do you come?), in a celebrated paper of 1963, stimulated interest in imported diseases, and encapsulated the principle of routinely taking a patient's *geographical history* as well as their clinical history.

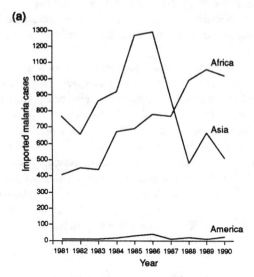

Source: Public Health Laboratory Service / R. Senior, 1992

Figure 14.5a Change in number of imported malaria cases from Africa, Asia and the Americas: 1981-1990

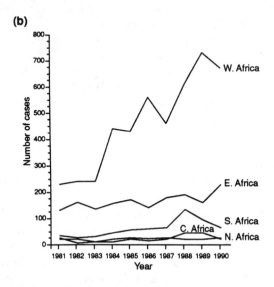

Figure 14.5b Malaria cases Africa-Britain: 1981-1990

The sources of pre-travel advice range widely over family practitioners (GPs), travel clinics, pharmacies, and general health service brochures, but many travellers are strongly influenced by the travel industry's own literature, and travel agents (TAs) are crucial links in the chain.

The Communicable Diseases (Scotland) Unit set up a pioneering telephone advisory service in the Scottish primary health care sector in 1975, and a travel information data base (TRAVAX) followed in 1982, making a data base nationally accessible (Cossar, 1988, 1992). A 1985 study in Scotland had shown that a minority (48%) of travellers surveyed had sought pre-travel advice, with travel agents (22%) being more frequently consulted than family doctors - despite the fact that the latter presumably knew their patients' medical histories, immunization records and life styles.

The work done at the CDSU in urging holiday companies to improve their holiday advice by paying for access to a health data base through telephone networking is an important development (Cossar et al, 1993a), but the comment that "specific health advice continues to be inconsistent, ranging from the mention of just one disease to tabular information", and that "some of the incorrect information given at best could give travellers a false sense of security and at worst result in their risking a preventable infection" offsets the improvement reported by the CDSU that the proportion of brochures carrying health information had increased between 1985 and 1992 (Cossar et al, 1993b) and has ramifications far beyond the glossy brochures concerned.

As the CDSU authors suggest, GPs and TAs occupy a key role in giving travel health advice, and the provision of effective advice can be shown to be "cost effective in terms of reduced hospital admissions, primary care consultations, laboratory investigations, specialist consultations, drug prescriptions, loss of working days and loss of vacation time due to potentially preventable illnesses" (Cossar et al. 1993a). The case for including high quality health information in all such travel literature seems unarguable.

Conclusion

Emporiatics, medical geography, and future tasks

Problems associated with travellers' health and travel medicine have come to the fore in recent decades with the unprecedented growth and variety of modern tourism enterprise, and the term *emporiatics* has been coined for this new field of enquiry.

In reviewing a hitherto fragmented or compartmented but necessarily multidisciplinary approach to safeguarding the health of individuals and ensuring the sustainability of tourism in potentially hazardous areas, it has become clear that applied medical geography might make a considerable, indeed an essential, contribution to both public health and development of the tourist sector in developing countries.

Obvious techniques might include the employment of traditional cartography and geographical information systems in producing maps of high, medium and low risk areas.

The parallels with mountain hazards mapping (United Nations, 1985) might be cited, but wider environmental risk assessment could become an integral part of the planning feasibility stage for tourism projects, and continue as a monitoring exercise, given the dynamics of disease and environmental change. Disease-risk maps of tourist development areas should become routine in the way that landscape epidemiology was used in the former Soviet Union in opening-up pioneer areas where the natural nidality of transmissible diseases - often viral zoonoses - was critical (Pavlovsky, 1966).

The historic links with geomedicine as part of military medicine and the conduct of war in such instances as the German Army's massive *Seuchen Atlas* of 1942-45 merit consideration, not least because infectious disease control and eradication remains a "war" against a microbial enemy. The publications of the Geomedical Research Centre at the Heidelberg Academy of Sciences, which spanned nearly four decades from 1952 and included the *World Atlas of Epidemic Diseases* and numerous geomedical monographs on tropical countries and tropic diseases, which grew out of this tradition (cf. Jusatz, 1983) constitute a resource which, in the author's view, has remained largely unexploited by anglophone scholars.

Writing in 1991, Gabriel Lee of the European Commission has noted that "the modern tourism sector and rapid developments in technology *require the same attention and professionalism, support and planning*, as has traditionally been applied... to agriculture and industry" (Lee, 1991). The italics are mine, but the words could provide a leitmotif and research agenda for the coming years.

In summary, many of the problems touched upon in this paper are the result of unplanned and unco-ordinated activities within the amorphous and acephelous tourist industry, of the narrowed focus of much contemporary medical education, or of widespread ignorance of tropical geography and the associated risks of disease importation and spread through tourist migration. Although the medical profession may be responsible for prevention through pre-travel immunizations and advice, and curative interventions when the system fails, the true costs are met by governments and individuals. The ultimate solutions will require fresh thinking about disease prevention on a global scale, but that in its turn will require close and hitherto unprecedented collaboration between researchers inside and outside medicine and those who direct or control the tourism industry worldwide.

References

Adams, A. R. D. and Maegraith, B. (1989). *Clinical Tropical Diseases* (9th Edition), Oxford: *Blackwell Scientific*.

Anderson, G.W. (1947). A German Atlas of Epidemic Diseases. *Geog. Rev.* 37.

Bender, R. J. (1993). Indien, ein touristisches Entwicklungsland?, *Die Erde* 124, 127-45.

Bernard, R. P. (1991). Incipient Thai Aids storm. International context, VIth Annual Meeting, Swiss Society for Medical Informatics, St. Gallen, pp. 9.

Black, J. (1992). *The British Abroad, The Grand Tour in the Eighteenth Century*, St. Martin's Press, New York.

Brendon, P. (1991). *Thomas Cook 150 Years of Popular Tourism*, Secker & Warburg, London.

Britton, S. (1991). Tourism, capital, and place: towards a critical geography of tourism, *Environment and Planning D; Society and Space*, 9, 451-78.

BTA/ETB (British Travel Authority/English Tourist Board) (1993). *Tourism Intelligence Quarterly, Research Services*, London.

Burgos, J.J., Fuenzalida Ponce, H. and Molion, L.C.B. (1991). *Climatic change predictions for South America*, Climatic Change 18, 223-39.

Cazes, G. 1992. *Tourisme et Tiers Monde: un bilan controverse. Les nouvelles colonies de vacances?* Editions de l'Harmattan, Paris.

Centre for Disease Control (CDC) (1992). *Health Information for International Travel*, U.S. Dept. of Health and Human Services, Atlanta, Georgia.

Cohen, M.N. 1989. *Health and the Rise of Civilization*, Yale Univ. Press, New Haven.

Cossar, J.H. et al. (1985). Illness associated with travel - a ten year review, *Travel Medicine International* 3, 1, 13-18.

Cossar, J.H. and Reid, D. (1989). Health hazards of international travel, *World Health Statistics Quarterly*, 42, 61-69.

Cossar, J.H., Reid, D., Fallon, R.J. et al. (1990). A cumulative review of studies on travellers, their experience of illness and the implications of these findings, *Journal of Infection* 21, 27-42.

Cossar, J.H. (1992). The Second Conference on International Travel Medicine. An update., *Scottish Medicine* 12, 1, 15-18.

Cossar, J. and Reid, D. (1992). Health advice for travellers: the GP's role, *British Journal of General Practice*, June, p. 260.

Cossar, J. H., McEachran, J. and Reid, D. (1993)(a), Pre-travel advice: are general practitioners and travel agents enthusiastic?, *Abstracts, World Congress on Tourist Medicine and Health*, 10th-15th January, 1993, Singapore.

Cossar, J.H., McEachran J. and Reid, D. (1993).(b), Holiday companies improve their health advice, *British Medical Journal* 306, 17 April.

Dawood, R. (1992). *Travellers' Health. How to Stay Healthy Abroad* (3rd Edition), Oxford University Press, Oxford.

De Schryver, A. and Meheus, A. (1989). International travel and sexually transmitted diseases, *World Health Statistics Quarterly* 42, 90-99.

Dieke, P.U.C. (1993). Tourism in The Gambia: some issues in development policy, *World Development* 21, 2, 277-26.

Domroes, M. (1985). Tourism resources and their development in the Maldive Islands, *GeoJournal* 10, 1, 119-26.

EIU (Economist Intelligence Unit) (1993). Travel and Tourism Analyst 2.

Epstein, R. (1993). Global village viruses, *Geographical Magazine* August, 32-36.

Fussell, P. (1980). *Abroad, British Literary Travelling Between the Wars*, Oxford University Press, New York.

Godlee, F. (1991). Health implications of climatic change, *British Medical Journal* 303, 1254-6.

Gotanegre, J.F. (1992). Le tourisme au, Rwanda: une émergence éphemère?, *Cahiers d'Outre-Mer* 45 (177), 21-40.

Gould, J.C. and Reid, D. (Organisers) (1982). *Travel, Disease and other Hazards, Symposium Report*, Proceedings of the Royal Society of Edinburgh 82A.

Green Flag International, (1993). *A Review of the Environmental Impact of the Travel Brochure Industry*, Cambridge.

Hansen, J., Fung, I. et al. (1988). Global climate change as forecast by the Goddard Institute for Space Studies three dimensional model, *J. Geophysical Research* 93, 9341-64.

Hellen, J.A. (1986). Medical geography and the Third World, in *Medical Geography: Progress and Prospect* (edited M. Pacione), pp. 284-332, Croom Helm, London.

Hohnholz, J. (Editor) (1984). *Thailand*, Thienemann Verlag, Stuttgart.

Holden, J.D. (1989). General practitioners and vaccinations for travellers, *J. Medical Defence Union*, March, pp. 6-7.

Howe, G.M. (1982). Does it matter where I go? In Gould and Reid (Eds) op. cit., pp. 75-96.

Hussey, A. (1989). Tourism in a Balinese Village, *Geographical Review* 79, 1, 311-25.

Jusatz, H.J. (1983). Geomedicine in Germany, 1952-1982, in *Geographical Aspects of Health*, edited N.D. McGlashan and J.R. Blunden, Academic Press, London.

Layton, M. and Bia, F.J. (1992). Emerging issues in travel medicine, *Current Opinion in Infectious Diseases* 5, 338-344.

Lazzarotti, O. (1993). Tourisme et Tiers Monde: de la connaissance au savoir geographique, *Annales de Geographie* 570, 181-7.

Lederberg, J., Shope, R.E. and Oaks, S.C. (Editors) (1992), *Emerging Infections: Microbial Threats to Health in the United States*, National Academy Press, Washington.

Lee, G. (1991). Lome and the tourism sector, *Tourism Management*, June, 149-151.

Lundberg, D.E. (1990). *The Tourist Business* (6th Edition), van Nostrand, New York.

Lundberg, D.E. and Lundberg, C.B. (1988). *International Travel and Tourism*, John Wiley, Chichester.

Maegraith, B. (1963). Unde venis?. *The Lancet* 1, 401-404.

McEachran, J. (1993). Pre-Travel health advice and the travel industry, unpublished BA dissertation, Dept. of Geography, University of Newcastle upon Tyne.

McNeil, W.H. (1977). *Plagues and Peoples*, Blackwell, Oxford.

Misato, N. (1991). The crossing of Japanese ODA and resort development, *AMPO Japan-Asia Quarterly Review* 22, 4, 34-6.

Neue Zürcher Zeitung, (1993). Drohende Aids-Katastrophe in Thailand, (special report), 184 (11 August), p. 3., Zurich.

Pasini, W. (1989). Tourist health as a new branch of public health, *World Health Statistics Quarterly* 42, 77-84.

Pavlovsky, E.N. (1966). *Natural Nidality of Transmissible Diseases. With Special Reference to the Landscape Epidemiology of Zooanthroponoses*, translated by N.D. Levine, University of Illinois Press, Urbana.

Pearce, D.G. (1984). Planning for tourism in Belize, *Geog. Rev.* 74, 291-303.

Pemble, J., (1991). From Grand to package tour, *Times Literary Supplement*, 15 January, p. 15.

Petty, R. (1989). Health limits to tourism development, *Tourism Management*, September, 209-12.

Peyrou, B. (1992). Le tourisme en Thailand, *Cahiers d'Outre-Mer* 45 (177), 55-76.

Phillips-Howard, P.A., Bradley, D.J., Blaze, M. and Hurn, M. 1988, Malaria in Britain. *British Medical Journal* 308, 245-296.

Phillips-Howard, P.A. et al (1990). Epidemic alert: malaria in travellers to West Africa, *The Lancet* 335, 119-121.

Ransford, O. (1983). *"Bid the Sickness Cease". Disease in the History of Black Africa*, John Murray, London.

Reiko, I. (1991). An army of Japanese tourists, *AMPO Japan-Asia Quarterly Review* 22, 4, 3-10.

Royal Geographical Society (1854-1938), *Hints to Travellers*, (1st to 11th Editions) London.

Senior, R. (1982). Hepatitis A and malaria. A danger to travellers' health, Unpublished BA dissertation, Dept. of Geography, University of Newcastle upon Tyne.

Steffen, R. et al. (1987). Health problems after travel to developing countries, *J. Infectious Diseases* 156, 1, 84-88.

The Economist, (1991). Travel and tourism supplement, March 23, pp. 3-26.

Troll, C. 1953. Ein Markstein in der Entwicklung der medizinischen Geographic, *Erdkunde* 7, 60-64.

Velimirovic, B. (1984). *Infectious Diseases in Europe. A Fresh Look*, WHO, Regional Office for Europe, Copenhagen.

Velimirovic, B. (1991). Health aspects of tourism in mountainous areas, *Travel Medicine International*, 9, 1, 11-17.

Velimirovic, B. (1991). Report on a meeting of the WHO Working Group on Immunisation of Tourists and Travellers, *Travel Medicine International* 9, 1, 83-85.

Velimirovic, B. (1991). Report on the Third International Conference on Tourist Health, *Travel Medicine International* 9, 1, 86-88.

Warren, K.S. and Mahmoud, A.A.F. (1990). *Tropical and Geographical Medicine* (2nd Edition), McGraw Hill, New York.

WHO (1986). *Tick-borne Encephalitis and Haemorrhagic Fever with Renal Syndrome in Europe. Report on a WHO Meeting, Euro Reports and Studies* 104, World Health Organization, Copenhagen.

Woodward, T.E. (1981). The Public's debt to military medicine, *Military Medicine* 146, 168-173.

Wyler, D.J. (1983). Malaria - resurgence, resistance and research, *New England J of Medicine* 308, pp. 875-8 and 934-40.

Zeiss, H. (Editor) (1942-45). *Seuchen Atlas,* Justus Perthes, Gotha.

Zimmermann, M. et al. (1986). Mountain hazards mapping in the Khumbu Himal, Nepal, with prototype map, scale 1:50,000, *Mountain Research and Development* 6, 1, 29 - 40.

15 Lifestyle and cardiovascular disease: Emerging problems of health development in the Third World

O. O. Akinkugbe

Summary

As developing countries strive to overcome the scourge of infectious diseases, a new range of diseases is beginning to emerge. Cardiovascular diseases, notably hypertension, constitutes a major component of these non-communicable diseases. They have in part to do with changes in lifestyle, including dietary habits, and seem destined to play a significant role in the profile of morbidity and mortality in these societies in the present decade and beyond.

A lot is known regarding risk factors in hypertension - excessive salt intake, obesity, lack of exercise, smoking, alcohol, stress and psycho-social factors. Ischaemic heart disease, though as yet relatively uncommon in the generality of these population, is beginning to be seen now and again in westernised, urbanised Africans. Its risk factors are almost akin to those of hypertension except that diet is more intricately involved.

It is important for every developing country to give both thought and time to investing in the cardiovascular health of its citizenry by not delaying any further programmes that anticipate or pre-empt the emergence of these "growing" diseases before they become major public health problems.

Introduction

There are striking contrasts both in the quantum and in the profile of cardiovascular disease as between industrial and developing nations. First, cardiovascular pathology (notably ishaemic heart disease and hypertension) remains the dominant feature of overall morbidity and mortality in the developed world, whereas these same conditions are as yet to constitute a major public health problem in third world countries, preoccupied as they are wih the burden of malnutrition and communicable diseases often compounded by ignorance (Fig.15.1)

As developing nations become emancipated and take on certain characteristics of socio-economic development, lifestyle and ecological changes become evident and the health profile undergoes some remarkable transformation. The example of Singapore is a classic case in point. In the four decades since 1948 its mortality emphasis has shifted from infection to cancer and cardiovascular disease. The cardiovascular profile of developed and developing countries is illustrated in Figure 15.2.

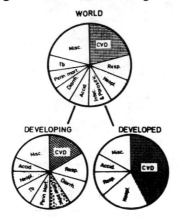

Figure 15.1 Global causes of mortality

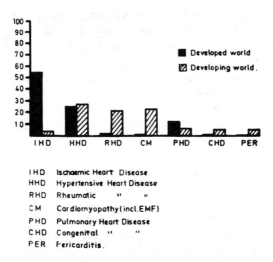

IHD	Ischaemic Heart Disease
HHD	Hypertensive Heart Disease
RHD	Rheumatic " "
CM	Cardiomyopathy (incl. EMF)
PHD	Pulmonary Heart Disease
CHD	Congenital " "
PER	Pericarditis.

Figure 15.2   Profile of cardiovascular diseases in the developed and developing world context (percentages indicate share of cardiac pathology for relevant environment)

Even in countries in which the quiet transformation is already taking place there are different cardiovascular profiles. In most of Asia and the Far East (Padmavati and Shestra, 1978) for instance, the major cardiovascular conditions are in the order of rheumatic heart disease, hypertension, ischaemic heart disease, and cor pulmonale. In Central and South America (PAHO 1982) it is hypertension, rheumatic heart disease, cardiomyopathy, (including Chagas disease), ischaemic heart disease and pulmonary hypertension. In Africa (Akinkugbe & Nicholson ,1991) however, the order of prevalence is hypertension, rheumatic heart disease and the cardiomyopathies. In the African setting, ischaemic heart disease remains much of a curiosity, particularly in rural communities.

Non-communicable disease encompasses a wide range of largely unrelated conditions, listed below for convenience:

- Hypertension (high blood pressure)
- Ischaemic heart disease (heart attacks)
- Diabetes mellitus
- Sickle cell disease
- Cancer
- Smoking-related conditions
- Occupational diseases
- Road traffic accidents
- Allergic states

It is impossible to address all these conditions in this exercise and for the purpose of this particular presentation I will focus on hypertension, ischaemic heart disease and cardiomyopathy. Passing references will be made to rheumatic heart disease (as it is a communicable disease) insofar as lifestyle changes affect its prevalence.

Hypertension

Four decades of intensive clinical, pathological and epidemiological studies of blood pressure in Nigerians have resulted in the following basic observations (Akinkugbe & Ojo 1969)

(i)   One in every 10 to 15 Nigerian adults is hypertensive

(ii)   Less than a third of those that have it are aware of the fact

(iii)   Less than a third of those who are aware are under any form of treatment

(iv)   Less than a third of those under treatment are adequately controlled

(v)   Uncontrolled hypertension often leads to such consequences a stroke, heart failure, kidney failure, visual impairment and may precipitate or aggravate heart attacks.

(vi)   The blood pressure increases steadily with age (Fig. 15.3) but there is a very small percentage of the community in whom this rise with age is hardly

179

perceptible, and in whom hypertension and its devastating consequences are distinctly uncommon.

It has long been recognised that lifestyle has profound effects on the behaviour of the blood pressure in particular and on the genesis and outcome of cardiovascular disease in general in any community. These influences are sometimes referred to as "risk factors" and for hypertension they include:

Excessive salt consumption
Obesity
Physical inactivity
Alcohol abuse
Stress and psycho-social factors.

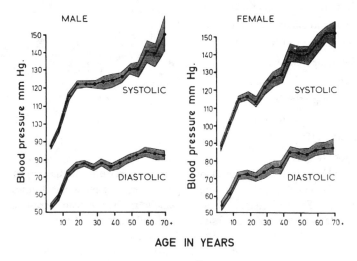

Figure 15.3   Rural study of mean arterial pressures (Eruwa - Nigeria)

Any of these predisposing risks compounded by such additional factors as advancing years and a strong family history make the emergence of hypertension almost inevitable.

The mere rise of blood pressure in the individual does not by itself presage the presence of target organ damage. Hypertension may thus be present for a long time before its untoward consequences become clinically manifest. This is why the condition is sometimes referred to as "the silent killer", and why attention to the risk factors enumerated above may delay or at best prevent the onset of complications. In classic studies of migrant communities in many parts of Africa it has been observed, for instance, that movement from a rural, preliterate environment to an urban setting with implications for salt intake, stress, alcohol abuse and sedentary habits associated with unemployment almost invariably lead to a rise in blood pressure and an increased incidence of hypertensive complications.

It is pertinent here to refer to one "stressor" that is known on the North American continent to be consistently related to elevated blood pressure. This is the so-called "life-style incongruity" or "John Henrysm" that measures the discrepancy between social class position and social class behaviour. In the setting of a developing country like Nigeria its equivalent would be an attempt to maintain a lifestyle that exceeds the individual's ability to increase their rank or social status.

Ischaemic heart disease (IHD)

Coming now to ischaemic heart disease a major risk factor is the presence of hypertension, but is complemented by:

- − Dietary fat intake
- − Cigarette smoking
- − Diabetes

It is known that the risk of a heart attack increases progressively with a total cholesterol above 150mg/dl and that a 40mg/dl increase in total cholesterol doubles that risk. Similarly, with tobacco, two cigarettes a day are worse than none at all, and twenty worse than ten.

The prevalence rate of IHD in Nigeria (Pobee, 1979) is less than 2% of the total number of cardiovascular diseases, compared to 20% in the developed world. Comparative mortality figures as percentages of death from cardiovascular diseases are 4% and 60% respectively. The reason for this marked contrast is neither genetic nor racial since the incidence of IHD in American Blacks, Caribbeans and in Indians in East, Central and Southern Africa is relatively high.

One of the best indicators of overall risk of IHD is the relative concentration of specific "lipoprotein" levels. The total cholesterol, high density lipoprotein ratios are higher in high than in low income groups. Indeed these values and serum cholesterol concentration in many professionals resident in urban centres in developing countries approximate to values in industrialized communities. And this is why heart attacks are becoming increasingly manifest in this particular group.

Conclusion

What lessons can we now draw from the foregoing account of risk factors in hypertension and in ischaemic heart disease? The old African saying seems pertinent here, that you look carefully at the twig sticking out of a tree well before you get to it so as to avoid its injuring your eye. It captures admirably the essence of prevention.

Primordial control measures can be integrated, at little extra cost, into any comprehensive primary health care (PHC) programme. Whether at the village level, the health post, health centre or regional hospital level, the basic approach to control is the same:

- Increasing public awareness of the hazards and consequences of these two conditions
- Screening at every opportunity
- Training suitable health personnel to measure blood pressure and recognise the early symptoms of IHD
- Regular surveillance of affected individuals and specific vulnerable groups
- Health education of the community regarding risk factors.

The limited resources and competing claims for health development in many third world countries have worked hardship on the effective implementation of primordial and primary preventive strategies. One of the risk factors amenable to control through habit, agricultural and economic policy legislation and appropriate health education techniques is cigarette smoking. There is as yet no concrete proof that most countries in the developing world are addressing themselves meaningfully to ways of stemming the tide of this growing scourge.

Of all the major cardiovascular conditions afflicting third world communities, rheumatic heart disease lends itself most readily to preventive measures (D'Arbella 1978) Primary prophylaxis will not be feasible until the epidemiology of streptococcal infection in childhood and adolescence is well recognised and until environmental protection programmes are mounted to control the spread of infection.

With respect to cardiomyopathy (Falae et al 1982) so little is known about its aetiology et al. that it is not possible to prescribe preventive measures to combat this peculiar form of heart disease.

It is a sad reflection of our times that not many countries in Africa today, nor even in the rest of the developing world, have a coherent and well-ordered programme for the control of cardiovascular diseases.

Nigeria is happily in the forefront of developing nations in Africa that do, for it put in place some two years ago a *National Task Force for the Control of Non-Communicable Diseases*. By doing this it is overtly giving thought and action to the prevention of a range of conditions that may not as yet constitute a serious threat in our midst, but whose effects are nevertheless so striking as to compromise the quality of life, means of livelihood of individuals, cohesion of families and productivity of communities. The 16-member committee has set out to define the extent and complexity of the NCD problem in the Nigerian context and

- identify risk factors
- promote greater awareness of NCD in general
- formulate a suitable programme for the detection, effective control and management of these conditions

- use all information gathered to design a satisfactory strategy for prevention
- train health officials at all levels in the proper methods of recognition of these diseases.

Any country that proceeds in this logical and visionary manner is investing wisely in the future of its citizens by anticipating the almost inevitable emergence of non-infective cardiovascular disease and doing something positive to prevent them, or at least diminish their untoward consequences.

This presentation has deliberately excluded consideration of management of the overt complications of hypertension and ischaemic heart disease, as indeed other types of cardiovascular disease resulting in heart failure, kidney failure, strokes and sudden death in developing world communities. Development of these complications are in effect manifestations of our inadequacies to deal effectively with precipitating or aggravating risk factors. But it must be remembered that even where these complications arise the natural history (or clinical progression) may be markedly influenced by the individual's lifestyle, dietary habit and socio-economic circumstances. Constraints in the Nigerian setting often include the sheer cost of medication, the growing challenge of procurement, availability and genuineness of the drugs and delays in patient hospitalisation.

References

Akinkugbe, O.O. and Ojo O.A. Arterial pressures in rural and urban populations in Nigeria. Brit. Med. J. (1969), 2, 222-224.

Akinkugbe, O.O., Nicholson G.D., and Cruickshank, J. Kennedy. (1991). "Heart Disease in Blacks of Africa and the Caribbean". In: Elijah Saunders (ed.) *Cardiovascular diseases in Blacks*. ed., Cardiovascular Clinics. Philadelphia, F. A. Davis Co. p. 377-391.

D'Arbella, P.G. 1978. Rheumatic Heart Disease and Infective Endocarditis - the problem in cardiological practice in Africa. In: O.O. Akinkugbe, (ed.) *Cardiovascular disease in Africa* Basel Ciba-Geigy, pp. 266-274.

Falase, A.O., Sekoni, G.A. and Adenle, A.D. (1982). "Dilated cardiomyopathy in young adult Africans - a sequel to infection". *Afr. J. Med. and Medical Sc.* 11,1.

Padmavati, S. and Shestra, N.K., (1978). "Problems of cadiovascular disease in Asia and Oceania". Internat. Congress Series No. 470. *Excerpta Medica.*

PAHO Scientific Publications Health Conditions in the Americas 1977-80. (1982). No. 427

Pobee J.O.M., (1979). "A view of Cardiovascular disease on the African continent". *Cardiovascular Epidemiology Newsletter* 26 23

Part IV
WOMEN AND HEALTH

Introduction

B. Folasade Iyun

There has been unprecedented growth in the production of literature on the marginaliza-
tion of women and deprivation of children derived from indices of good health that
originate from mothers of young children in Third World Countries.

This phenomenal growth owes its momentum basically to the current world economic
crises and in particular the biting health side effects of the structural adjustment programmes (SAP) imposed on many Third World countries by the World Bank and the
International Monetary Fund (IMF). For all this literature not to be self-defeating, more
concrete evidence beyond the dry medical demographic and other socio-economic figures
must be articulated for the identification of reasonable and practical efforts that can be
made at local, national, and international levels to reduce health risks and problems of
women and indirectly children in order to promote their health status in the face of current
development processes.

The key research issue is how to understand the effects of existing economic crisis,
social transition and near environmental collapse of many developing countries as they
affect the most vulnerable groups - mothers, the elderly women and young children across
cultures and across areas. Thus, this section of the book focuses on some aspects of this
issue. Even though the literature on gender issues is on the increase, the three papers touch
on key aspects of women's health to fill some of the gap in the literature.

The paper by Soyibo and two others focuses on the effects of the World Bank-assisted
agricultural development projects (ADPs) on the quality of life of women in Oyo North
of the former Western Nigeria, now Oyo State. One of the lessons learnt is that the ADPs
regard women as part of the household and benefits so accrued by their spouses would
"trickle down" to them. The ADPs appear not to have enhanced the economic viability
of the women in the enclave compared with women living in adjoining (control) areas.
However, the former are better off in respect to access to agricultural inputs. Even though
they made better use of immunization, ante- and post-natal services, they were still more

they made better use of immunization, ante- and post-natal services, they were still more conservative in the use of family planning (FP) services. By implication the quality of their life has not much improved by acceptance of new agricultural technology by their spouses.

The second paper by Omoluabi centres on the issue of child survival as it hinges on the physical and biological assaults experienced by their mothers. The author painstakingly explains the effects of housing and living conditions, in particular seasonal variability in food supply and adverse environmental conditions on the weight-velocity (child growth) of young children despite the attention accorded maternal education in the literature. According to the author, studies of a period of relative survival chances can go a long way in guiding decision makers in the Third World in the bid to reduce infant and child mortality.

The last paper by Udegbe examines the role of traditionally enjoyed extended family system support by elderly women in the prevailing economic circumstances in Oyo State, Nigeria. The author demonstrates the current health status of elderly women by their perception of life satisfaction, depression using appropriate index measurements for Nigeria.

Nearly all the study of elderly women indicated insufficiency of basic needs. Women with mixed support exhibited relatively better health status than those with only family support and the level of depression was higher among elderly urban women. The author advocates for government intervention to alleviate the problems of the elderly instead of the assumed adequate family support since meeting the needs of the female elderly in particular, place a lot of strain on care givers under the existing economic crises in the Third World.

These papers further illustrate that the priority task facing local, national and international organizations and agencies on improvement in the health status of women and children is in the right direction. Sustainable development must take care of women and children health predicaments.

16 Agricultural development projects and women's quality of life in Nigeria: A case study

Adedoyin Soyibo, B. Folasade Iyun and T. Ademola Oyejide

Introduction

In recent times improvement in the status of women has been a priority task for many national and international organizations. Such efforts to improve the situation of women seems to have followed the concerted drive of the United Nations in proclaiming the period 1976-1985, the International Decade for Women's Equality, Development and Peace. Since this historic proclamation, various agencies have embarked upon projects to improve the quality of life of women particularly in developing societies. Even though not much seems to have been achieved in these societies, certainly the awareness about the seriousness of the situation for a majority of nations has increased. Also, as a follow-up, some international organizations including the World Bank now insist on devoting a given proportion of fund meant for rural development in the Third World countries be directed at improving the quality of life of women and children. One of such programmes is the Agricultural Development Projects (ADPs) in Nigeria.

This paper is part of a project evaluation study of the impact of ADPs on the status of rural women in Nigeria. This aspect of the study specifically focuses on the impact of the ADPs on the quality of life of women in the project area. However, the topic requires analysis of the differentials between the quality of life of the rural women in the programme and the non-programme (control) areas, using former Oyo North Agricultural Development Project (ONADEP) and adjacent areas as a case study.

Methodology and concept of women's quality of life

This study is an impact assessment study. There are at least three approaches to assessing policy impacts (Murphy, 1985). Before/after Comparison Approach in which the value of a situation X at the beginning of the programme at time t_1, (Xt_1) is compared with the value at time t_2, the end of the programme (Xt_2). Here $Xt_2 - Xt_1$ measures the impact.

Expected Comparison Approach in which the value of situation X at the end of the programme (Xt_2) is compared with a targeted value say X'. The deviation X' - Xt_2 measures the assessed impact. With/without Comparison Approach which measures the change between the value of the situation with the programme as its end (Xt_2) and the value of the situation with the programme as its end (Xt_2) and the value of the situation if there was no such programme time t_2 (Yt_2). The impact assessment index in this case is Xt_2 - Yt_2. The with/without comparison methodology is similar to the use of controls in experimental and medical sciences.

The methodology adopted in this study is the With/Without Comparison Approach. It involves comparing activities of women in the programme area with those of women in adjoining non-programme control areas. In the larger study, activities of women were also compared with those of men in the programme area.

A total of 733 households were selected by the use of a multi-stage sampling procedure. First, a list of all participating villages/settlements was compiled and arranged in alphabetical order for the selection of the study area. The number of wards in the selected villages/settlements was used as weighting. Then, the number of households to be interviewed was selected by using existing households as weighting. Finally, the specific households to be interviewed were selected by the use of a systematic random sampling technique with a sampling interval of ten households. In each selected household, every female of age 15 and above was interviewed, while only male heads of households were interviewed in the programme area. In the control area, a similar procedure was followed to interview females aged 15 and above.

The main purpose of this paper is to assess the impact of ADPs on the quality of life of women in the programme area. In general the ADPs are meant to improve the productivity and standard of living of farm families. However, Boserup (1970) does not believe that technical change in agriculture, as implied in the implementation of the ADPs, improves the status of women. According to her, the status of such women often tends to remain more or less static. The problem is that the ADPs regard women as part of the households and that benefits accruing to men "trickle down" to women. The main hypothesis is that the development processes in sub-Saharan Africa has tended to marginalise, demote or downgrade rural women in the subsistence sector (Boserup, 1970; Stamp, 1989).

The quality of life of women is multidimensional. Accordingly, several attempts have been made at constructing compound indices of female quality of life. By and large, indices often adopted include female literacy rate, life expectancy and a measure of fertility (number of births per woman) (Andrews, 1982). In this connection, high fertility is treated as a negative measure.

It is also known that becoming pregnant again soon after giving birth roughly doubles the risk to the life and health of both mother and children. Hence, there is a link between quality of life and acceptance of contraception by women (Grant, 1986).

Women are also said to expend at least 9% of their caloric intake on water collection (Isely, 1981), therefore a more accessible water supply can release time and energy for other household tasks such as nurturing children. Besides this, women benefit from access to potable water by a reduction in the morbidity from water-related and water-borne diseases suffered by children under 2 years old in particular.

It is also known that women improve their lives by their own informed decisions and actions taken on certain issues such as acceptance of family planning and control of resources among others.

Therefore, this study adopts the use of certain indicative indices such as income, access to potable water, health services, educational institutions, power to make certain decisions, among others, to assess the quality of life of the women living in the former ONADEP enclave.

Main findings of the study

Socio-economic-demographic characteristics of respondents

Table 16.1 shows the economic activities engaged in by the respondents. It is of interest to note that a much less proportion of the women in the control area engage in farming. However, they are still less represented in non-primary activities. When the proportion in sewing and school is compared with those from the control area, it seems that some of them avoid agricultural activities and concentrate more on trading in agricultural products which probably come from the farms of their spouses.

When the educational achievements of the respondents were considered, it is obvious that those outside the programme area possess better educational status in respect of secondary and post-secondary education in particular (Table 16.2). Since education enhances the quality of life of individuals, it is likely that this factor may be a significant determinant in the quality of life of the two locations; it is already noted that they are less represented in tertiary activities.

Next, the analysis considers the purposes of performing some economic activities so as to be able to identify differentials in the welfare of the women. Table 16.3 shows the level of subsistence in the performance of certain activities in both the programme and control areas. In all the selected activities as depicted in Table 16. 3, the women in the control area appear to be more viable economically. With the exception of crop farming, they have the tendency to aim more at earning cash in the performance of various economic activities compared with women in the programme area.

For instance 10-68.3% of the women in the control area indicated they were performing activities for cash only for crop farming and food processing. On the other hand, only 2.6-44.7% of women in the programme area stressed the economic factor as the most significant reason for performing the selected activities. Even in respect of crop farming and food processing where the ADPs were meant to enhance their productivity, less than 5% of them are involved for economic venture. In this respect, it seems the ADP has not enhanced the economic viability of these women, in spite of its presence.

In the same vein the yearly earnings of the two groups of women from all sources were compared in spite of their inherent problems of reliability. Table 16.4 confirms that women in the programme area appear to earn less than those in the control area. For instance while 54% of women in programme area stated they earned up to N1000 (US$125.00 at the time of research), just about 31% of the control women earned as little. Indeed, about threefold (21.8%) of women in the control area earned over N3,000 (US$375.00) compared with those in the programme area (7.3%).

Table 16.1
Job done most of the time by female respondents

Job	Programme area		Control area	
	No. of women	%	No. of women	%
Farming	293	17.3	323	30.1
Trading in agricultural products	403	23.8	121	11.3
Trading in manufactured goods	246	14.5	119	11.1
Food processing	75	4.4	37	3.5
Craft making	120	7.1	25	2.3
Food vending	72	4.3	36	3.4
Sewing	139	8.2	43	4.0
Housewife	33	1.2	22	2.1
Schooling	172	10.2	206	19.2
Job seeker	67	4.0	67	6.3
Pensioner	3	0.2	6	0.6
Others	39	2.3	63	5.9

In the programme area 74.3% of the women stated that they kept separate accounts from their husbands as against 83.7% in the control area. When asked to compare their earnings with their spouses, Table 16.5 indicated that 80.2% felt their husbands earned much more highly compared with almost 90% in the control area. However, more women

Table 16.2
Highest educational qualification

Education	Programme area		Control area	
	No. of women	%	No. of women	%
1. No school	805	48.23	403	37.66
2. Adult education	127	7.61	43	4.02
3. Koranic education	95	5.69	26	2.43
4. Some primary	134	8.03	47	4.39
5. Completed primary	189	11.32	98	9.16
6. Some secondary	150	8.98	142	13.27
7. Completed secondary	115	6.89	171	15.98
8. Above secondary	53	3.18	134	12.52
9. Others	1	0.06	6	0.56
Total	1,669	100.00	1070	100.00

confirmed they are better off than their spouses in the control area, even though Table 16.5 gives the impression that more women in the programme area appear to be better off than their spouses. However, when asked about ownership of private buildings, slightly more of them have put up their own buildings compared with their counterparts in the control area. Nonetheless, they seem relatively deprived of farm land against the control area as indicated in Table 16.6. Also slightly more women (40.0%) in the control area enjoyed the assistance of house-help compared with 35.0% in the programme area.

As indicated by Andrews (1982), certain demographic attributes of females can be treated as positive or negative measures of their living conditions. For this purpose, some selected maternity characteristics of the respondents were chosen for comparative analysis. Table 16.7 depicts the selected attributes.

Considering the parity of the respondents 81.2% of them enjoyed low to medium parity as against 84.4% in the control. Likewise a higher proportion of them (17.4%) compared with 14.5% in the control area are likely to experience the negative effects of high fertility rates. With respect to child mortality, the control area also appears to fare better. For instance, 26.7% of the respondents in the control area said they had lost at least one child compared with 35% in the programme area. It can be observed that child mortality appears to be relatively higher in the programme area compared with the control area. Moreover,

Table 16.3
Purposes of performing certain economic activities

Education	Programme area		Control area	
	No. of women	%	No. of women	%
Keeping poultry:				
Cash only	73	4.9	62	10.0
Consumption only	528	35.3	216	34.8
Both	894	59.8	343	55.2
Food processing:				
Cash only	39	2.6	48	6.9
Consumption only	573	38.6	155	22.2
Both	871	58.7	494	70.9
Trading in agricultural products:				
Cash only	203	13.6	137	20.5
Consumption only	238	16.0	61	9.1
Both	1,049	70.4	472	70.5
Trading in manufactured goods:				
Cash only	352	26.8	264	49.0
Consumption only	210	15.7	55	10.2
Both	778	58.1	220	40.8
Craft making:				
Cash only	569	44.7	301	68.3
Consumption only	151	11.9	28	6.5
Both	544	42.7	112	25.4
Crop farming:				
Cash only	74	4.4	38	3.5
Consumption only	289	17.1	111	10.4
Both	1,103	65.3	471	43.9
Activity earning most income:				
Farming	397	27.8	419	55.6
Secondary	1,023	71.5	331	13.9
Don't know	10	0.7	4	0.5

Table 16.4
Yearly income from all sources

Income	Programme area		Control area	
	No. of women	%	No. of women	%
Up to ₦500	331	23.88	72	9.69
₦501 - ₦1000	420	30.30	163	21.94
₦1001 - ₦2000	337	24.31	190	25.57
₦N2001 - ₦3000	189	13.64	155	20.86
₦3001 - ₦5000	74	5.34	112	15.07
Above ₦5000	78	2.02	50	6.73
Don't know	7	0.51	1	0.13
Total	1,386	100.00	743	100.00

Table 16.5
Comparison of income with husband's income

Income	Programme area		Control area	
	No. of women	%	No of women	%
He earns higher income	828	80.23	503	89.82
He earns about the same	116	11.24	34	6.07
He earns much less	19	1.84	12	2.14
He earns a little less	6	0.58	4	0.71
Don't know	63	6.10	7	1.25
Total	1032	100.00	560	100.00

Table 16.6
Ownership of property

Ownership		Programme area		Control area	
		No. of women	%	No. of women	%
Farm plot	Yes	624	41.68	493	55.46
	No	873	58.32	396	44.54
Building	Yes	175	10.70	100	9.64
	No	1,460	89.30	937	90.36

Table 16.7
Maternity characteristics of female respondents

Characteristics	Programme area		Control area	
	No. of women	%	No. of women	%
Parity				
1 - 3	404	33.2	238	36.8
4 - 6	585	48.0	308	47.6
7 and above	212	17.4	94	14.5
Child mortality				
Ever lost	438	35.0	175	26.7
1 - 2	350	71.9	144	70.6
3 - 4	90	18.5	32	15.7
5+	47	9.7	13	6.4
None	815	65.0	480	73.3
Length of use of FP (in months)				
Up to 12	104	6.2	43	4.0
13 - 24	118	7.0	94	8.8
25 - 36	71	4.2	81	7.6
Over 36	42	2.5	69	6.7
No specific opinion	1299	76.8	746	69.6

more women in the programme area seem to be less specific on length of use of family planning (76.8%) compared with 69.6% in the control area.

Impact of access to selected amenities and services

Table 16.8 indicates that the ADPs must have enhanced greatly the access of the women in the programme area to agricultural inputs. They appear much favoured in respect of access to important agricultural inputs such as bank credit, cooperative farming except use of tractors. On the other hand, Table 16.9 indicates that they are not much better than women outside the programme area when possession of selected household items and social amenities that should reduce some of the burden of the women are considered. Indeed the possession of some of these items make life more comfortable for individuals. In a few cases women in the control area are better off, in particular the proportion of their households possessing radio, room with ceiling, borehole, kerosene stove etc. Nonetheless, they seem to be slightly better off in possession of wells and piped water from dams.

196

Impact of utilization of social services

In order to assess the quality of life of women living in the former enclave of ONADEP, some selected health care services were compiled. For instance, attendance at ante-natal clinic before child birth and presence of a trained person at birth effectively protect child and mother. Table 16.10 depicts the selected health care services. It can be observed on the table that the women in the programme area made better use of maternal immunization service as well as ante-natal and post-natal clinics compared with those in the control area. They also showed better patronage of child health care services such as immunization against tuberculosis (BCG), measles and health education on child nutrition. Yet, they appear to experience higher child mortality.

Table 16.8
Percentage of women using modern agricultural techniques

Technique	Programme area	Control area
Fertilizer	60.7	57.5
Improved seed varieties	30.5	17.5
Improved poultry varieties	29.9	9.8
Chemicals	30.4	31.2
Animal feeds	13.7	11.1
Irrigation	10.6	4.1
Tractors	35.7	39.7
Harvesters	22.4	2.6
Bank Credit	5.4	2.1
Cooperative farming and fishing	9.2	3.9

Considering utilization of family planning services, their patronage is almost double (50.1%) that of the control area (27.1%) as indicated in Table 16.10. A further analysis of types of family planning services utilized by the respondents revealed a cautionary note on the performance of the women in the programme area. Even though these women reported much higher rates of use of family planning services, most of them (42.5%) were actually utilizing some inefficient methods (Oni, 1986; Birdsall and other, 1987) such as abstinence and withdrawal. On the other hand, women in the control area patronize more of modern and very efficient methods (19.1%) of family planning. The result of this aspect of the analysis seems to suggest some conservative attitudes on the part of women in the programme area towards family planning. This attitude may not be unconnected with their observed relatively higher fertility and mortality rates already observed in their population.

Table 16.9
Percentage of household with selected amenities in the areas of study

Social amenity	Programme area	Control area
Kerosene stove	73.9	79.9
Iron bed	80.5	77.4
Foam mattress	78.7	80.8
Dining table	37.8	33.9
Wall/table clock	23.9	40.8
Baby cot	12.5	14.0
Pit latrine	32.0	37.0
Radio	54.0	68.5
Chairs with arm rest	57.7	58.7
Wall calendar	74.6	83.5
Room with ceiling	87.9	75.8
Windows in rooms	94.1	89.4
Water closet	0.1	0.9
Household well	0.0	0.8
Pipe-borne water from dam	2.3	0.6
Tanker from outside village	0.1	0.5
Borehole	1.4	6.3
Well	77.0	61.9
Asbestos roof	6.6	8.3
Plastic container for storing water	9.8	14.3
Metal drum	1.8	2.8
Well dug after programme implementation	31.9	32.6
Block wall materials	23.1	20.4
Personal building	10.7	9.6

Impact on participation of women in decision-making at the household level

The ability or freedom of the woman to make personal decisions on certain issues somehow engenders some political power for her and therefore promotes her capability in controlling her resources. The women were asked about whose responsibility it was to take decisions on some specific issues at the household level.

It is interesting to note that women in the programme area appear to be taking relatively more independent decisions (wife-led) on relative to live in household, household purchase, house decoration, pregnancy with the exception of child spacing compared with women in the control area (Table 16.11). This observation, however, is still consistent with our earlier suggestion that women in the programme area appear more conservative compared with those in the control area in respect of family planning (child spacing). This aspect of their weakness further suggests that their quality of life has not improved much or been influenced by the acceptance of a new agricultural technology by their spouses.

In spite of the previous observation, the majority of the women in the enclave still appear to leave a lot of decisions to be taken on their behalf by their spouses (husband-led, Table 16.11) compared with how they fare in joint responsibility. This result probably implies that the subordination of women is probably the same in both ADP and control areas considering the proportion of the latter that confirmed sole responsibility of heads of households (mostly husbands) in decision making.

Conclusion

In order to evaluate the impact of the ADPs on the quality of life of the affected rural women, an attempt has been made to compare their performance or attributes with women in the adjoining area, since no baseline information is available in the former ONADEP enclave. For this purpose certain indicative indices were selected. These indices relate to the earning power, access to some social amenities, some demographic attributes as well as the level of the women using their ability to make certain decision.

In general, not much improvement has been noted in the quality of life (status) of the women in the programme area. Their performance in respect of yearly income appears to be lower than women in the adjacent areas, even though they enjoy better access to potable water. However, they still appear more conservative in particular with respect to the types of family planning methods utilized by the women. Since they appear to patronize mostly abstinence which is very inefficient, this probably explains why they have relatively higher fertility rates, whilst child mortality is also higher among them.

It appears the ADPs have made them more dependent of their spouses, as a large number of them appear to have been deprived of their farm lands while they now trade more in agricultural products "purchased" from the farms of their spouses. In this respect it may appear the ADPs have made them more subordinate to their spouses compared with women in the non-programme area. If anything the result is indicative that their quality of life is rather static, as not much of improvement has been observed in the present study. It is therefore necessary that in planning agricultural development projects, the needs of women should be taken into consideration explicitly.

Table 16.10
Percentage of women using selected health services

Health services	Programme area	Control area
Antenatal care	57.0	40.1
Postnatal care	54.7	39.2
Maternal immunization	52.3	37.7
Ever-used family planning (FP)	25.6	26.2
Currently using FP	50.0	27.1
Currently using very efficient methods*	5.4	19.1
Currently using moderately efficient methods**	2.5	4.5
Currently using inefficient method***	42.5	4.1
No specific method mentioned	9.9	10.6
Child immunization	52.5	37.8
Child nutrition	49.7	31.9
BCG immunization	23.5	20.6
Measles	18.8	13.3

*Pills, IUD, injectables, sterilization

**Condom, foam tables

***Abstinence, withdrawal

Table 16.11

Level of participation of women in decision-making at household level

Type of decision	Programme area		Control area	
	No. of women	%	No. of women	%
On relation who lives in household				
Self	783	51.7	266	25.8
Husband alone	51	3.4	25	2.4
Self and Husband	439	29.0	207	20.0
Head of household alone	233	15.4	470	45.5
Self and head of household	9	0.6	32	3.1
Others	1	0.1	33	3.2
Household purchases				
Self	421	25.2	119	7.1
Husband alone	376	22.5	224	13.4
Self and husband	656	39.3	251	15.0
Head of household alone	161	9.6	405	24.2
Self and head of household	45	2.7	33	2.0
Others	12	0.7	24	1.4
On house decoration				
Self	729	43.5	242	22.9
Husband alone	293	17.5	55	5.2
Self and husband	458	27.3	355	33.7
Head of household alone	136	8.1	345	32.7
Self and head of household	47	2.8	31	2.9
Others	12	0.7	27	2.6
On pregnancy				
Self	285	17.1	40	4.3
Husband alone	608	36.6	220	23.4
Self and husband	579	34.8	332	35.3
Head of household alone	151	9.1	99	10.5
Self and head of household	28	1.7	28	3.0
Others	12	0.7	221	23.5
On child spacing				
Self	292	17.6	288	20.7
Husband alone	605	36.4	44	0.7
Self and husband	576	34.7	275	22.9
Head of household alone	149	9.0	85	9.1
Self and head of household	27	1.6	27	2.9
Self and head of household	27	1.6	27	2.9
Others	12	0.7	219	23.4

A. Soyibo, B. Folasade Iyun and T. Ademola Oyejide

Acknowledgement

The authors gratefully acknowledge that this research is part of a larger study funded by a grant from the Rockefeller Foundation.

References

Andrews, A.C. (1982). 'Towards a status of women index', *Professional Geographer,* 34, (1) 24-31.

Birdsall, M. and Chester, L.A. (1987). 'Contraception and the status of women: what is the link? *Family Planning Perspectives* 19; (1) 14-17.

Boserup, E. (1970). *Woman's Role in Economic Development.* New York, St. Martin's Press.

Grant, J.P. (1986). *The State of the World's Children,*' UNICEF, 54-55.

Isely, R.B. (1981). The Relationship of Accessible Safe Water and Adequate Sanitation to Maternal and Child looking forward to the Drinking Water and Sanitation Decade', *Water Supply and Management,* 5, 417-424.

Oni, G.A. (1986). 'Contraceptive Knowledge and Attitudes in Urban Ilorin, Nigeria'. *Jour. of Biosoc. Sci.,* 18, 273-283.

Stamp, P. (1989). 'Technology, Gender and Power' Technical Study 63e, Funded by the International Development Research Centre and the Rockefeller Foundation.

17 Child health in Ondo state: Seasonal fluctuation of weight velocity

Elizabeth Omoluabi

Summary

In a situation of high infant and child mortality associated with infectious and parasitic diseases, the death of a child is most often the end result of a series of illnesses, each of which weakens the child's resistance. It has been observed that growth faltering is one of the processes linking disease to child death. The study of variations in growth velocity of children points at critical periods in a child's life when his morbidity and mortality risks are high. Seasonal variation in growth velocity is analyzed in terms of exposure to certain diseases as well as changes in nutritional inputs. In this study children aged from one month to forty months in a rural area were visited twice during the dry season and twice during the rainy season. At each visit they were weighed and their arm circumferences taken. The rainy season appears to be a period of high risk for children in rural areas. Multi-staged surveys are recommended in the study of child health.

Child health and health infrastructure

At the time of independence there were two health care systems in the West Africa: the traditional system, and the modern or allopathic system. The latter was proving inadequate to cater for the health care needs of the growing population. Consequently, one of the first activities of the governments of the newly independent countries was to embark upon grandiose health care projects, which involved the construction of large hospitals in which heavy and expensive technology was concentrated.

At the end of the 70s most of these countries were faced with two problems: not only was the inherited health care system not efficient, it was also becoming a very heavy burden to bear in the face of rapid population growth. The collapse of this elaborate system was imminent (Mosley, 1985). Certain authors have observed that the rate of mortality decrease had slowed down or even stopped (Gwatkin, 1980) while others found no evidence associating any decrease in mortality with the activities of the health care services (Garenne *et al.* 1985). If today specialists on the subject all agree that there is a decline in mortality all over Africa, the gap between West Africa, and the rest of the world is increasing faster than before (Hill, 1989). In the special case of Nigeria, available data shows that within the last ten years childhood mortality has increased from 144 deaths per 1000 births in 1982 to 192 deaths per 1000 in 1990 (FOS and IRD 1991).

Modelisation of mortality and child health

Many authors have tried to examine the problem of morbidity and its relationship with child mortality. Considering the low levels of infant and child mortality in developed countries it is evident that the survival potential of a human child is very high indeed. The level of mortality in developing countries shows that this potential is far from being attained. The reduction in survival potential "is a direct consequence of physical and biological assaults on the individual which may have their origin with the mother even before conception, and which continue during pregnancy, childbirth and throughout early childhood" (Mosely, 1985).

Although nobody interested in the subject will dispute the argument that the immediate environment holds the key to an explanation of child survival, the very limits of this environment are more or less fixed by different disciplines. Studies in the social sciences have concentrated on the socio-economic aspects of morbidity and mortality: maternal educational levels, father's education, income, area of residence, etc. Purely demographic studies have concentrated on mother's age, parity and birth intervals. Medical sciences have tended to lay more emphasis on the medical aspects of disease and death: prevalence and incidence of disease, reaction to different therapeutic measures, evaluation of risks related to biological factors. Below is a short discussion of the areas of interest and the theoretical framework of research in the social sciences.

The role of maternal education, evidence and controversies

The World Fertility Surveys have provided useful information on female fertility as well as childhood mortality in many West African countries. An important point raised by these surveys is the inverse relation between a mother's level of education and the survival of her child. Children of educated women, especially if the latter have completed secondary education, have much higher survival chances than children of illiterate mothers. Although these surveys were unable to explain the mechanisms governing this relationship, in attracting attention to the socio-economic characteristics of the parents, they thus reaffirmed at the national level, conclusions already reached at regional levels by smaller studies. Some studies which have addressed themselves to this problem have shown that maternal education works at three different levels: it influences the socio-economic level of the household, it governs a mother's attitude and influences her behaviour on issues relating to the health of her child.

The inverse relation between the economic level of the household and problems of over-population, hygiene and morbidity is well documented (Okediji, 1973; Ho, 1982). However, a study in northern Nigeria has recorded higher morbidity rates among children of "wealthier" households (Longhurst, 1984). Despite the ambiguity surrounding the subject, it has been shown that half of the decrease in mortality experienced by educated women compared to illiterate women is due to the higher economic level of the former's households (United Nations, 1985). Educated women tend to marry men of equal or higher qualifications and also tend to have highly paid jobs compared to illiterate women.

After adjusting for the effect of the economic level on childhood mortality however, (Orubuloye *et al.* (1975) found a residue which they attributed to the difference in the attitude and behaviour of educated women. The latter have a less fatalistic attitude towards childhood disease, have more confidence in modern medicine, and have more autonomy in decision making where the health of their children is concerned (Orubuloye and Caldwell, 1975). The difference in behaviour between the two groups of women is even more striking than their attitudes. Educated women spend more time alone with their children (who tend to have fewer mother substitutes than other children of illiterate mothers living in a traditional rural setting). They also take their children to hospital for consultation more regularly.

Place of residence

Maternal education has received more attention than other socio-economic variables because it is easy to study, but many studies of child mortality in West Africa while recognising the explanatory power of maternal education, accord as much importance to other factors, like the housing location and living conditions (Dackam N'Gatchou, 1987). Within the group which shares this opinion one finds authors who persistently question this apparently negative relationship between maternal education and childhood mortality, especially when other socio-economic factors are controlled. It is the case in Bobo-Dioulaso where (M'backe and van de Walle, 1987) found that the level of post-neonatal mortality was explained more by housing quality, income levels and clinic attendance than by female education alone.

Ethnic group

A study of countries in sub-Saharan Africa has shown that a mother's ethnic group plays an important role in her child's survival. In some of them maternal education falls behind the ethnic group in explaining childhood mortality. It is the case in Cameroun, where the ethnic groups with the lowest childhood mortality levels are by no means the ones with the highest levels of education (IFORD., 1989).

The choice of mortality as an outcome variable by demographers is borne out of their lack of familiarity with biomedical research methods and tools. Infant mortality has the added advantage of being easily measurable and at a lower cost than most anthropometric or morbidity measures. Changes in infant and child mortality provide a clear indicator of change in the state of health of the country or region (van de Walle, 1991).

For the past fifteen years relatively robust estimates of mortality in childhood have been made from the World Fertility Surveys and more recently, the Demographic and Health Surveys conducted in many countries all over the world. This filled a vacuum at a time when information at an international level was sparse. Numerous comparative studies were carried out which situated countries according to their levels of mortality in childhood. It was not surprising that industrialised countries were in the low mortality group and developing countries in the other camp. What was interesting, however, was the heterogeneity found among the developing countries. While the life expectancies of sub-Saharan countries remained the lowest on earth, those of Sri Lanka and Kerala (India), at 70 years, are almost in the same category as developed countries (Caldwell, 1991).

Beyond this interesting and thought-provoking observation, traditional demography is at a loss over identifying and explaining the dynamics of these disparities.

Limitations of mortality estimates

Mortality estimates are based on censuses or surveys covering a large number of people, and consequently they can easily be generalized, unlike measures of growth or morbidity. This characteristic is also, unfortunately, the major source of weakness in demographic research because enough attention is not paid to the minute micro-level linkages between phenomena observed at a macro level. An infant mortality rate calculated for a country does not give any indication of high risk periods in a child's life. It applies for periods ranging from one year to five years. In practical terms, most mortality studies cannot indicate at what period of the year a child's survival chances are lowest. Consequently, the results of these studies, though of undisputed theoretical value, cannot efficiently guide decision makers in their bid to reduce infant and child mortality. The discovery that children of educated women have higher survival chances than those of illiterate mothers has no immediate practical significance in a country where less than 20 per cent of women have secondary education. However, the knowledge that childhood diseases are more severe at certain months of the year for every child may help to increase the vigilance of care givers during these periods of risk. Our data show that the rainy season is a particularly risky period for child survival in Nigeria. This confirms similar observations in Senegal (Rosetta, 1988) and in Gambia (Rowland et al; 1988). Morbidity studies like ours are important in providing the link between our knowledge of child mortality and the conditions surrounding it. These studies provide the substance from which to interpret mortality data.

The survey: subjects, methods and materials

The survey on family health-seeking behaviour and child health was aimed at collecting information on the socio-cultural environment of child health in Nigeria. It took place between February 1991 and May 1992.

The sample consisted of all women of parity two and above whose youngest child was below 45 months at the beginning of the survey. There were 299 women and 395 children at the beginning of the study but at each subsequent visit this number has been reduced mostly by emigration but also by mortality. Each child received five visits in the 15 months of the study. At each visit, the mother provided information on the health status of the child. She was asked if her child had diarrhoea, fever or cough in the last two weeks and what actions she took in this regard. The child was then weighed and the arm circumference measured. Weights were taken with a TALC lightweight spring balance graduated to 17kg and mid-arm circumference with an insertion tape obtained from TALC, England. Apart from the health status, which is updated at each visit, certain themes pertaining to child health were studied. The main instrument for the study consisted of a series of questionnaires, one of which was administered at each visit. As much as possible the same interviewers were recruited at each visit in order to reduce measurement errors. The major part of this chapter draws on the preliminary results of the first four visits.

Survey location

Akure Local Government Area (administrative district) was chosen for the study. The proximity of Akure, the capital of Ondo State introduced the problem of defining a rural area. It was impossible to find a village large enough to have the 250 children necessary for the study. The sites which had a suitable population size were urban in nature with a high proportion of non-agricultural activity, proximity of an important hospital, presence of secondary schools and other government institutions. Ondo State, like most predominantly Yoruba-speaking areas is highly urbanised. Forty percent of the population lives in an urban area. A compromise was finally arrived at by selecting 4 villages and 9 small hamlets all less than 25 kilometres from the capital and located in three enumeration areas demarcated by the National Population Commission.

The population of Akure Local Government Area is estimated at 276,574 (Ministry of Health, Ondo State, 1989). This should be viewed with caution as it is a projection from the 1963 census figure to which a growth rate of 2.5% per annum was applied up to 1981 and then it was increased to 3.2%. Fortunately, a census has just been undertaken which will, we hope, update the present figures.

Background characteristics of respondents

In this section we shall study the background characteristics of the mothers and the children in the sample. In the discussion of maternal variables, attention will also be paid to certain characteristics of their households in order better to situate these women and their children.

Age of mothers

In this rural population many mothers were incapable of giving a satisfactory figure when asked 'how old are you?' or 'in what year were you born?' Where the woman gave a figure for age, rounding was frequently encountered. There was a clear attraction for figures ending in '0' or '5'. In one case out of five a mother's age had to be estimated. The historical calendar drawn up for the purpose of aiding in recall proved largely ineffective as many of the women are recent immigrants who came to work on the cocoa farms with their husbands. In most surveys in rural populations errors in age declaration are often encountered. Generally one of the numerous methods available (Gendreau *et al.*, 1985) is chosen to smooth the data. However, since our sample omitted women with less than two live births, as well as those among them who did not have a young child below four years old, smoothing of the age distribution using traditional techniques would have introduced more errors than were originally present in the data.

Table 17.1
Percentage distribution of mothers by age (Akure survey 1991)

Age of woman	percentage	Number of women
under 25	20.1	59
25-29	27.2	80
30-34	26.2	77
35-39	13.3	39
above 39	12.9	38
missing	0.3	01
Total	100.0	294

The relatively young age of the women in the sample is due to the fact that they are at the peak of childbearing. The age distribution of the mothers is shown in Table 17.1 above. Less than 9% of the respondents were below 22 years old. This is to be expected with a median age at first birth of 20.5 years (DHS Ondo State p.25). The majority (87%) of respondents were, however, less than 40 years old. These women accounted for 86% of Total Fertility Rate in 1990 (DHS Nigeria, preliminary Report p.6). Average age of respondents was 30 years.

Marriage pattern

All the respondents were married and, but for one woman, living with their husbands at the time of our first visit. This does not in any way exclude the presence of single mothers in the population. However, they were automatically excluded by the selection process, simply because they tended to have only one birth (their first). The older ones among them who were multiparous did not have a child under four years old. This implies that young women with more than one birth tend to stay with their husbands, especially when the youngest child is less than five years old.

The predominant marriage type is monogamy. Only 50 of the 294 respondents were in a polygynous marriage, which in most cases consisted of two wives. In general, the level of polygyny increases with age. It is highest among women above 34 years old. The practice of polygyny seems to be on the decline if present levels are compared with those of 1971 (Adepoju, 1979). This may be a temporary phenomenon associated with the present economic crisis. Also, a woman may be in a polygamous marriage one day and a monogamous marriage the day her co-wife abandons the matrimonial home. Polygyny is such a dynamic phenomenon that a proper study requires in-depth retrospective marriage histories of men and women (Tabutin, and Vallin, 1977).

Maternal Education

Table 17.2
Maternal educational levels

Year of education	Percentage	Number
0 - 2	36.4	71
3 - 6	37.4	73
7+	26.2	51
Total	100.0	195

About 36% of the women for whom information on education was available were illiterate. Another 37% can barely read or write with less than seven years of primary education. The proportion of women with secondary education in our sample (26%) is less than the Ondo State average of 35% calculated by DHS in 1986 but is closer to the national average (FOS and IRD, 1991).

Nutritional status of the children

Measurements of height for age were taken in Ondo State in 1986. They showed that 32% of children aged 6-36 months were stunted (i.e. 2 or more standard deviations below the WHO/CDC/NCHS reference). The weight for age of the same children showed that 28% of them were in a state of undernutrition. Children from rural areas were at a disadvantage compared to urban children.

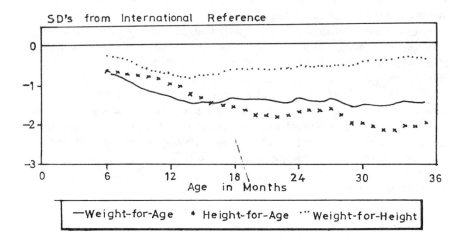

**Figure 17.1   Nutritional status of children age 6-36 months compared to interna-
tional reference. Source: Ondo State DHS, 1986**

Problems with international standards

Errors in age declaration render the use of international anthropometric standards delicate
in developing countries. In rural areas a child born in November may be said to be one
year old in February of the following year. The difference between 25 months and 36
months is often clearer in the mind of the researcher than that of the mother being
interviewed. Consequently, in the absence of an accurate civil registration system any
interpretation of anthropometric measurements in comparison with international standards should be done with caution. Multi-staged surveys with data to show the evolution
in weight of the same child can produce results which are easier to interpret in the Nigerian
context.

The second important variable to be aware of in the interpretation of anthropometric
measures is the season in which the measurements were taken. In rural West Africa,
existence is so regulated by the natural forces that people gain weight during the months
of relative surplus after the harvest and lose weight during the rainy season. This seasonal
fluctuation of weight velocity may be an important factor in growth faltering among
Nigerian children.

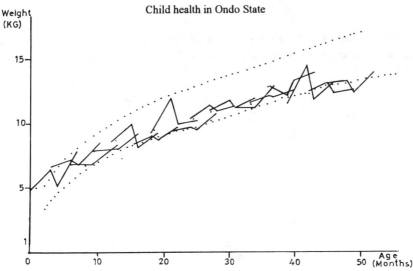

Figure 17.2   Seasonal evolution of mean weight for age in Akure

Fig. 17.2 shows the average weights of children in the sample in three month age groups. There is an evident increase in weight by age (P<0.001). There appears to be no significant difference in weight between boys and girls of the same age. This graph shows that the children are well on the "road to health" traced by the World Health Organization. The "road to health" is a section of a growth chart, the upper limit of which represents the 50th percentile of the WHO recommended standard weight for age for boys, and the lower limit, that of the 3rd percentile for girls. A child is said to be in good health when his growth curve falls within this limit. In studies where it has been possible to measure children from birth, African children appear to be at a nutritional advantage up to the age of six months when compared with any international standard (Rowland *et al.* 1988). Our results confirm this observation.

From the age of twelve months the weights of the children in the sample begin to fall close to the lower limit of the "road to health". This is the critical area in the growth curve of the African child. It corresponds with the period when breast milk is no longer a sufficient source of nourishment. The child is already beginning to sample adult food and is being confronted with the bacteria and viruses in his environment. More often than not the mother is already carrying the next pregnancy, which will oblige her to hasten the weaning process. The importance of studying child growth is borne out of the fact that growth is a sensitive indicator of adverse environmental conditions. One of the first signs of malnutrition and infection in children is growth faltering. Here, the child is not being compared with a well-fed American or European standard but with himself. There are 16 age groups covering ages 0 to 50 months. Each curve has four points representing the average weight of the age group at each of the visits. The first visit was in February 1991, the second in May, the third in July and the fourth in October of the same year. The first and last visits took place during the dry season while the May and July visits corresponded with the rainy season. Consequently, it was possible to record with relative accuracy the seasonal evolution in the weight of each child. At the individual level weight was significantly correlated with season (P<0.001)). The period between May and July 1991 was a period of weight loss for almost all of the children in the sample as shown by the sudden dip of the curves at the third visit. Three months later, in October, most of the children had recovered and were slightly heavier than at the beginning of the study.

Weight velocity and seasonal fluctuation

Weight velocity is calculated for a certain period by comparing a child's weight at the beginning and at the end of the period by the time interval. It expresses the average weight gained (or lost) by a child per day during the period under study. The results of weight velocity by age are shown in Fig. 17.3.

The weight velocity for each period is represented by a bar which is linked to that of the subsequent period by dotted lines. The bars below the zero line show the average amount of weight loss in grams/day during the rainy season, while the bars above represent weight gain. The graph shows an initial period of weight gain followed by weight loss and at the third interval there is a second period of weight gain. The important observation here is that more than 85% of the children lost weight at the same time, without any conscious deliberate action on the part of older members of the household responsible for their care.

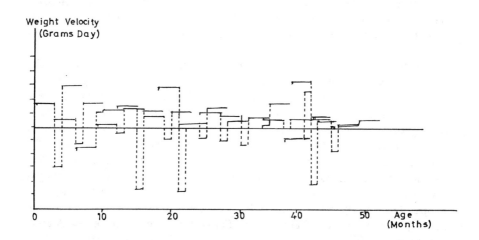

Figure 17.3 Average weight velocities of age groups of Akure children

Arm circumference and recent illness

Arm circumference is a very sensitive indicator of recent weight loss and it consequently, can point to recent illness in a child.

Table 17.3
Values for mean arm circumference (millimetres) in the presence or absence of illness.

Date of visit	Absence of illness	Presence of illness
February	143	141
July	144	137
October	148	139

In most cases of recent illness the mid-arm circumference was below 137mm. There is no significant change in the arm circumference during the rainy season for children who have not had an episode of illness (143 and 144mm). Children who were ill at the time of our visit or recovering from an illness episode consistently have lower arm circumference values. The mid-arm circumference of children who have not had an illness episode increased by as much as 4 mm between July and October which, when compared with the period between February and July, indicates that growth around the month of July was slow. While in February there was hardly any difference in arm circumference between children who had at least one episode of illness and those who had not, by October the gap which declared itself during the rainy season had widened considerably.

Conclusion

It would appear from the above that the rainy season is a particularly risky period which accentuates the difference in survival chances of children. The rainy season is a period of peak agricultural activity for the rural population. It is also a period when food is relatively scarce and the rural population dips into its reserves for nutritional inputs. In such situations of hardship children are often the first victims. The work load during the rainy season may be responsible for a certain reduction in the vigilance of mothers. They may react less quickly to illness in young children simply because they are more tired than usual. Yet it is the same rainy season which is responsible for the proliferation of malaria parasites as well as the contamination of drinking water which lead to child illness. Since we only asked if the child had been ill within the two weeks preceding each visit, it is impossible to know if there are more disease episodes during the rainy season than during the dry season. However, it would appear that disease episodes are more severe during the rainy season as children are already weakened by the nutritional constraints imposed by the rainy season. The reduction in nutritional inputs at the household level implies that the mother's production of milk is reduced, resulting in a reduction in a suckling child's resistance to disease.

The results of this study show that special attention should be paid to child health during the rainy season. Care givers should be encouraged to be more vigilant at this period, which represents a period of high risk to all children below five years old.

References

Adepoju, A., (1979). 'Introduction' in Adeokun, L.A. (ed.) 1971-75 National Survey on Fertility, Family and Family Planning Phase 1: South Western Nigeria, DSS monograph no.1, University of Ife.

Adeokun, L.A., (1983). 'Nature, Evolution and Organisation of Health Intervention Programmes in Nigeria', Presented at the Seminar on The Influence of Health Policies on the Future Evolution of Mortality, INED, Paris.

Caldwell, J.C., (1990). 'Introductory thoughts on Health Transition' in Caldwell *et al.* (eds) *What we know about Health Transition: the cultural, social and behavioural determinants of health* xi-xii.

Dackam N'gatchou R., (1987). Causes et Déterminants de la Mortalité des Enfants de Moins de cinq ans en Afrique Tropical. Doctoral Thesis in Demography, Université de Paris I.

FOS, Lagos and IRD, (1991). 'Nigeria Demographic and Health Survey 1990, Preliminary Report'.

Garenne M., Diop, I.L., Contrell P., (1985). 'Politique de santé et mortalité au Sénégal 1960-1980,' in Vallin & Lopez, La lutte contre la morti: I. influence des politiques soiciales et des politiques de santé sur l, évolution future de la 4: mortalité; Paris, PUF.

Gwatkin, D.R. (1980). 'Indicators of Changes in Developing Country Mortality Trends: the end of an era'? *Population and Development Review*, 6, 4 615-644.

Hill, A. (1989). 'La mortalité des Enfants: Niveaux actuel et Évolution depuis 1945, in Pison G. *et al.*, Mortalité et société en Afrique au sud du Saharan, Paris, PUF

Ho T.J., (1982). 'Measuring Health as a Component of Living Standards', *World Bank Working Paper* No. 15.

IFORD, (1989). 'Analyse Descriptive des Rapports entre quelques Variables Biologiques, Demographiques et Socio-économiques et la Mortalité Infantile à Yaounde', EMIJ III Tome III.

International Conference on Primary Health Care, Alma Atta, (USSR), 6-12 September (1978).

Longhurst, R., (1984). 'The Energy Trap: Work, Nutrition and Child Malnutrition in northern Nigeria'. *Cornell International Nutrition Monograph Series* No. 13

M'backe C., van de Walle E., (1987). 'Les Facteurs Socio-Économiques et l'influence de la Fréquentation des Services de santé, in Pison G. *et. al.*, Mortalité et Societe en Afrique au sud du Saharan: Paris, PUF. 67-87.

Mosley, W.H., (1985). Les soins de Santé primaries peuvent-ils réduire la mortalité infantile? Bilan critique de quelques Programmes Africains et asiatiques, in Vallin, J., Lopez, A., 'La lutte contre la mort: l'influence des politiques sociales et des politiques de santé sur l'évolution future de la mortalité. Paris, PUF.

Okediji, F, (1973). 'Caracteristiques Socio-Économiques et attitudes à l'égard des problèmes de santé Publique dans l'état de l'Ouest au Nigéria: le cas d'Ibadan', in Caldwell, J.C.,, (ed) Croissance Démographique et Évolution socio-Économique en Afrique de l'Quest.

Orubuloye, I.O., Caldwell, J.C. (1975). The Impact of Health Services on Mortality: a Study of Differentials in a Rural Area in Nigeria'. Population Studies 29 257-272.

Rosetta, L., (1988). 'Seasonal Changes in the Physical Development of Young Serere children in Senegal, Annals of Human Biology: 15, (3) 179-189.

Rowland, G.M., Rowland, S., Cole T., (1988). 'Impact of Infection on Growth of Children in an Urban West African community' Am. J. Clin Nutr, 47: 134-8.

Tabutin, D. and Vallin J., (1977). 'La nuptialité' in 'Source et Analyse des Données Démographiques Part 3, II INED-INSEE-MINCOOP-ORSTOM, Paris.

United Nations, (1985). Socio-economic Differentials in Child Mortality in Developing Countries, Department of International Economic and Social Affairs, New York.

van de Walle E., (1990). 'How do we define Health Transition?' in Caldwell J., Findley S., Caldwell P., Santow G., Cosford., Braid J., Broers-Freeman D., (eds) What we know about Health Transition: the Cultural, Social and Behavioural Determinants of Health. Vol. I The Australian National University.

18 Current adjustment patterns of elderly Yoruba women and their health implications

I. Bola Udegbe

Summary

This paper examined some current patterns of adjustment and some health implications. 706 elderly women (mean age 60.8 years) were interviewed in 21 local government areas of old Oyo State. Results indicated that many elderly women are currently engaged in economic activities partially or fully to support themselves. Using regression analysis, results showed that geographical location, perceived progress, life satisfaction and health were significant predictors of depression. When the independent variables were regressed on perceived health educational level of children, working due to necessity, geographical location, depression and life satisfaction were significant predictors of perceived health. Finally, the type of family support showed a significant effect on perceived health.

Introduction

Over the years, there has been a gradual shift in the care of the elderly in Nigeria. Traditionally, the elderly live within the extended family system in which their support is the sole responsibility of their kin. In other words, in the pre-Western Nigerian societies the economic, social and emotional needs of the elderly were met through these informal social networks. However, urbanization, rural transition, migration and industrialization have brought about changes to the status of the elderly (Udegbe, 1990). Unlike in the developed countries such as the U.S.A., with Old Age Survivor's Insurance (OASI), and the U.K., with social security, there is an absence of social security for the elderly with the exception of employers' pension schemes, which accrue only to those retiring from salaried employment, usually in the informal sector. Unfortunately, owing to male bias in education and employment only a negligible proportion of elderly women are entitled to such benefits.

At the present day Nigeria, with problems of inflation and economic crisis, the status of the elderly is changing. Adult children find it difficult to meet the needs of their elderly parents (Togonu-Bickersteith, 1988). This poses a challenge in adjustment for the elderly. As Udegbe (1991) noted, 92% of rural elderly Yoruba women engaged in economic activities for sustenance. Indeed, many receive only partial or inadequate support from their kin. This paper therefore aims to examine some current adjustment patterns among elderly Yoruba women and their health implications.

Methodology

Sample and subjects

This research focused on elderly women who resided in the old Oyo State (now new Oyo and Oshun States). The sample selection was purposive because only elderly women over 54 years were included in the study. For a representative sample of the State, 50% (21) of the local government areas were randomly selected from a list of all the local government areas in the State. 706 elderly women were used in the study. Of these, 35% were resident in urban areas while 65% were resident in rural areas. Their ages ranged from 55 years to 105 years (mean = 60.8 years). Their educational level ranged from none to university. 71% were married, 14% widowed, 11% divorced or separated and 1% single.

Instrument

An interview schedule containing both open- and close-ended questions was used to elicit information from respondents. As part of a larger study on predictors of adjustment in old age, the questions asked of respondents included those on personal demographic characteristics, social support, life satisfaction, perceived progress (independent variables), depression and perceived health (dependent variables).

The personal demographic characteristics included variables such as respondent's age, income, educational level, marital status, age of husband, number of children, number of years married and widowed and geographical location. In addition, the number of wives the husband has, the position of the respondent among the husband's wives, the educational level of the first and second children were also solicited from the elderly women.

Respondents also provided information about the number of religious associations they belonged to, their involvement in such activities (i.e. frequency of attendance per week), their major worries, obstacles and economic activities.

On social support system, respondents were asked if they solved problems related to feeding by depending on themselves (i.e. working, property), family (children and husband) or mixed sources. Other variables were life satisfaction, perceived progress and health. Two indices of health were used in this study: depression and perceived health status. Because this study involved interviewing women in Yoruba language, it was envisaged that too many questions may increase interpretation errors. Furthermore, since previous studies (e.g. Higgins and Dicharry, 1990) have provided evidence for cross-cultural differences in acceptability of some items on scales, those that were to be perceived as unacceptable were deleted. Thus, few items were taken from valid and reliable scales. Life satisfaction was measured by 3 items on life satisfaction inventory (Neugarten *et al*; 1961). The life satisfaction index measured on a 5-point Likert-type response format is a valid and reliable measure which has been used in studies in Nigeria among aged illiterate Nigerians (Togonu-Bickersteth, 1986). Three items from Zung's (1965) depression scale were also used to measure depression on a 5-point agree-disagree format. The reliability and validity of the Zung scale in Nigeria has been demonstrated by Jegede (1976). Perceived progress in this study was measured by three items which required each individual to indicate if she considered that she was happier, more comfortable, and financially better off now than when she was younger. Perceived health status was measured on a 5-point (poor - very good) Likert-type scale.

Procedure

Trained research assistants visited the randomly selected 21 local government headquarters and approached various heads of households to obtain permission for conducting interviews with the elderly women. Although many of them feared political and legal repercussions, their fears were allayed by briefly explaining the purpose of the research. Participation was voluntary and the interviews were conducted in the Yoruba language. Altogether 735 women were interviewed but responses from 29 women were rejected, due mostly to incompleteness of the interview schedule. Consequently, a net sample of 706 was used in the study.

Result

90% of the respondents indicated that they still engaged in economic activities, ranging from farming (12%), petty trading (43%), business (16%), civil service (17%), to other activities in the informal sector (4%). When asked why they worked, 12% reportedly did so to relieve boredom, 9% out of interest, while a majority (70%) did so to have money for sustenance. However, 65% indicated that they would still be working even if they had money to feed, while 35% indicated that they would not. The monthly income of the elderly women in this sample ranged from none to N3,000 ($\overline{X} = 453.20$, SD = 422.78). Almost all the women indicated that their income was not adequate for their basic needs.

When asked how the women solved the problem of feeding (a basic need) 35% indicated that they depended solely on themselves, 30% on their family and 35% on both family and themselves. Perhaps an indication that many elderly women still expect to depend solely on family is the fact that the well-being of their children was the most important thing the women worried about (39%). Other sources of worry were financial problems (14%), health (11%) and basic survival (6%).

To what extent can depression and perceived health be predicted by the independent variables in the study? The results of the regression on the independent variables are presented in Table 18.1 below.

The table shows that geographical location, life satisfaction, perceived progress and perceived health were significant predictors of depression (the betas were 0.09, 0.35, 0.14 and 0.11 respectively). Altogether, all independent variables accounted for 30% (P<0.001) of variance in depression.

The extent to which the independent variables predicted perceived health is reflected in the betas presented in Table 18.2. The results show that education of the first and second children, working due to necessity, geographical location, depression and life satisfaction are significant predictors of perceived health. The amount of variance in perceived health accounted for by all the variables in the equation was 19% (P<0.001).

Table 18.1

Regression of depression on predictor variables

Variables	Beta
Age	-0.03
Husband's age	0.09
Wives' position	0.03
Number of wives	0.01
Widowed years	0.05
Education	-0.04
Children (number)	-0.03
Education (1st child)	0.04
Education (2nd child)	0.08
Co-inhabitants (number)	0.03
Dependants (number)	0.0
Working due to necessity	0.00
Religious groups (number)	0.08
Religious groups (attendance)	-0.08
Income	-0.04
Geographical location	0.09*
Perceived progress	0.14***
Life satisfaction	0.35***
Health status	0.11**
R^2	0.30***

*P <0.05, ** P<0.01 ***P<0.001
Note: Low score reflects high depression.

Two separate one-way ANOVA were carried out to examine the differences in depression and perceived health between those who had self-, family- and mixed support in solving problems of feeding. Results presented in Table 18.3 show that while depression did not have any significant effect, perceived health differed among the three groups $(F(2,645) = 2.32$, n.s. and $F(2,679) = 406$, $P<0.05$ respectively). A post-hoc analysis showed the direction of the difference observed in perceived health. Those who had mixed support exhibited relatively better health status than those in the family support group. There were no significant differences between the self-support and the mixed- or family support group.

Table 18.2
Regression of health on predictor variables

Variable	Total B
Age	.09
Husband age	.02
Wives position	-.05
Wives (no)	.04
Education	.00
Children (no)	.04
Depression children	.04
Education (1st child)	.15**
Education (2nd chiild)	.15**
Necessity work	-.12**
Religious gp (no)	.04
Religious gp (att)	.01
Income	.08
Geographical 10c.	.08*
Depression	.09*
Personal progress	.07
Life satisfaction	.19***
R^2	.19***

*P<.05	**P<.01	***P>.001

Discussion and conclusion

The most important predictors of depression among the elderly women were geographical location, perceived progress, life satisfaction and perceived health. The higher their perceived health, life satisfaction and perceived progress, the lower the depression experienced. An important predictor, which was geographical location, suggests that there exist significant differences in the levels of depression of elderly women in rural and urban

Table 18.3
Summary on one-way ANOVA for depression and perceived health

Sources	df	MS	F	df	MS	F
	Depression			Health		
Between group		2.00	22.76	2.32[a]	2.00	7.37
Within group	647	9.81		679	1.80	4.06*
Total	647			681		

a n.s.   *P < .05

Table 18.4
Scheffe test for differences among means of the three groups on health

Group	Support type	1	2	3
1	Self			
2	Family	a	a	
3	Mixed	a	*	

* Pair significant at .05

a Pair not significantly different

areas. Specifically, the level of depression was higher among the urban elderly. This finding is consistent with Togonu-Bickersteth's assertion (1988) that there is an increasing number of elderly destitutes in Nigerian urban centres . These destitutes, who moved to urban centres in their younger days, had either lost contact with relatives in rural areas or had relations who had reneged on their obligations to them.

The higher the respondents' level of life satisfaction and the educational attainment of their children, the better they perceived their health status. This is probably because higher educational attainment of children increases the probability of fulfilling filial obligations effectively (Togonu-Bickersteth, 1988). The results also indicated that poorer health status was higher among respondents who worked due to necessity and lived in urban centres.

While there are no significant differences in the level of depression of the three groups of women with different social support for feeding, it was found that those who had mixed support had moderately better health status than the family support group. Furthermore, studies which have focused on self-efficacy as a mediator of stress perceptions have suggested that low perceived self-efficacy may be detrimental to appraisals and effective coping with stress (e.g. Abler & Fretz, 1988; Holohan & Holohan, 1987). Generally, the findings suggest that moderate amount of activity is beneficial to elderly women; however, working in response to harsh economic conditions may be altogether harmful.

This research is not without limitations. First, a more in-depth study is needed in which more health indices rather than only self-reporting will be used. Secondly, the study only focused on elderly Yoruba women. The study should be expanded to other parts of Nigeria in order to see if the adjustment patterns and health implications change across ethnic groups.

In conclusion, the findings of this study suggest a need for government intervention to alleviate problems associated with aging. Although some women still depend solely or partially on kin support for sustenance, meeting the needs of the elderly poses a lot of strain on the care-giver and recipients. It seems likely that future adjustment of the elderly may become more difficult, due to rising inflation and economic crisis. Thus, intervention programmes would require more in-depth analysis into problems of the elderly and how best to help alleviate them.

Acknowledgement

The author gratefully acknowledges that this research was funded by a grant from the Social Science Council of Nigeria/Ford Foundation.

References

Abler, R.M. and Fretz, B. (1988). 'Self-efficacy and Competence: Independent Living Among Old Persons'. *Journal of Gerontology,* 43, 5133-5143.

Higgins, P.G. and Dicharry, E.K. (1990). 'Measurement Issues in the Use of Coopersmith Self-Esteem Inventory with Navajo Women. *Health Care for Women International,* 11, 251-262.

Holahan, C.K. and Holahan, C.J. (1987). 'Self-efficacy, Social Support and Depression In Aging: A Longitudinal Analysis. *Journal of Gerontology,* 42, 65-68.

Jegede, R.O. (1976). 'Psychometric Properties of the Self-Rating Depression Scale. *Journal of Psychology,* 93, 97-130.

Neugarten, B.L., Haughurst, R.J. and Tobin, S.S. (1961). The Measurement of Life Satisfaction. *Journal of Gerontology,* 16, 134-143.

Togonu-Bickersteth, F. (1986). 'Age Identification Among Yoruba Aged.' *Journal of Gerontology* 41, 110-113.

Togonu-Bickersteth, F. (1988). 'Aging in Nigeria: Current and Future Policy for Caring for the Elderly.' *Journal of Applied Gerontology,* 7, 474-484.

Udegbe, I.B. (1990). 'Supporting Older Women in Nigeria: Current Issues and Implications.' *Journal of Issues in Social Sciences* 1: 71-77.

Udegbe, I.B. (1991). 'Economic Activities of Rural Elderly Yoruba Women.' A Paper Presented at the Conference of the Ibadan Socio-Economic Group, July, 1991, Ibadan.

Zung, W.W.K. (1973). 'From Art to Science: The Diagnosis and Treatment of Depression.' *Archives of General Psychiatry,* 29, 328-337.

Part V
HEALTH CARE PROVISION IN A THIRD WORLD CONTEXT

Introduction

Elizabeth M. Thomas-Hope

Health care provision in any society reflects the nature of the political economy, the system of administration and management, personnel, technology and pharmaceuticals employed in the delivery of care, the people's concept of health, and the patterns of consumer behaviour in the utilization of the service. It is not surprising that no narrow intellectual discipline could adequately address a topic of such breadth or that policy decisions should be made without cognizance of the varied implications of the many aspects involved.

The ensuing group of papers in this section of the volume addresses a small selection of the issues that health care provision entails. It brings together perspectives of social science and medicine, and it raises issues on both the supply and the consumer sides of the provision. Each of these aspects are discussed in specific case studies which are important when one considers that it is only within the particular political economies, societal priorities and locational conditions that health care provision can be meaningfully discussed.

The first three chapters outline problems in the control of the use of drugs in Third World countries. This includes cross national comparisons of drug use, doctors' awareness of the International Network for the Rational Use of Drugs (INRUD), and the problems of irrational and inappropriate dispensing of drugs that occurs.

The next three chapters evaluate problems of health service provisions from the consumer perspective. The first of these highlights the low use of health centres in the case of urban Nepal. This contrasts with the following chapter which discusses the high use in urban Jamaica. The Jamaican case further raises the issue of severe financial constraints in maintaining a comprehensive system of health care and the occurrence of serious inequalities of access to facilities of some sectors of the population due to poverty, old age or problems of immobility. The issue of unequal access to health is further elaborated by a chapter on the variable success of immunization programmes for children in north western Nigeria. The variability in the benefit of the vaccine among the population is based not on inequality of physical accessibility to the provision but the unsuitability of the programme to those groups suffering material deprivation.

The final chapter draws attention to the issue of minority health needs. While women and the aged have become widely recognized as groups with specific needs over and above those of the general needs of the population, persons with disabilities have not been recognized in this regard. As a result, they have largely remained an invisible group in both the agendas for research as well as national and international policy.

Overall, this section draws attention to a number of the deficiencies and ineffectiveness of health care provision in various national contexts and examines different themes. In so doing, it is intended that some contribution may be made to the deeper understanding of the problems surrounding health care provisions in the Third World. The objective is that in turn this may assist in bringing about a greater appreciation of areas in which further research should be conducted and the attention of policy directed at both national and international levels.

19 Prescription for childhood watery diarrhoea in Nigeria: A comparison of pharmaceutical chemists and patent medicine shops

U. A. Igun

Summary

Based on a combination of open and confederates survey of one hundred and thirty-five pharmacies and patent medicine shops in Borno state in the north-eastern part of Nigeria, this study aimed at documenting and analyzing what retail pharmacies prescribe for childhood diarrhoea.

The study found that retail pharmacies in the overwhelming majority, routinely prescribed non-rehydration medications, such as antidiarrhoea, antibiotics and antimicrobial agents, for watery diarrhoea. Very few of the pharmacies (pharmaceutical chemists and patent shops) prescribed any form of ORT for watery diarrhoea.

The study examined the implications of this irrational use of drugs for watery diarrhoeal for diarrhoea control programmes, health development and resources allocation in the development of the country.

Introduction

Diarrhoeal diseases constitute a major killer of African children particularly in illiterate urban slum-dwelling families. In Nigeria, diarrhoeal diseases are the single most frequently reported illness among urban slum-dwelling children (Igun, 1982). One of the most important advances in technical knowledge about the management of diarrhoeal diseases in recent times, is the discovery that a solution of oral rehydration salts (ORS), can be used to treat dehydration caused by diarrhoea of any aetiology, in any age group (Merson, 1988).

The Federal Government of Nigeria started a programme to institute the use of ORT as the major prop of diarrhoea management in the country. In its ORT programme, the Federal Government adopted salt sugar solution (SSS) as the ORS to promote the home management of diarrhoea. This is now being actively promoted at all levels of the Nigerian health care system. Through the mass media, mothers and children caretakers are also being taught to prepare and use at home, the solution by combining one teaspoon of salt with ten teaspoons of granulated sugar in a pint (Nigerian beer bottle) of cooled boiled water.

Retail pharmacies are frequently and regularly used by populations in developing countries as outpatient clinics. Reports of such outpatient clinical practice by pharmacies are many in the literature from developing countries. Examples include van der Geest (1982); Mabadeje (1974); Igun (1987); Logan (1983); Haak (1988); Price (1989); Tomson and Sterky (1986); Wolffers (1987); Thamlikitkul (1988); Dressler (1982); Mitchell (1983); Ferguson (1981); Nichter (1983); and Sussman (1981).

These reports indicate that in most developing countries such as Nigeria, pharmacies play the role of outpatient clinics and are so recognized by the public, even though the legal position is against such practice. In these countries, the retail pharmacies are usually the first point of contact between patients and the modern medical system. In many such countries, they represent for many communities, the only source of modern medical care accessible to the majority of the people.

Consequently, any positive or negative effects of their practices are likely to have far reaching implications for health development in these countries. Their prescribing practices may by contributing either positively to attempts to solve the diarrhoea problem or negatively and hence exacerbating it, complicating it and creating new problems. Their practices may also have serious implications for these countries' attempt to achieve a more rational use of drugs and pharmaceuticals.

The study

The data reported in this paper was generated as part of a larger study of retail pharmacies prescription for childhood diarrhoea, funded by the Applied Diarrhoea Disease Research (ADDR) project of Havard University (grant 064).

The study aimed centrally to document the prescribing practices of retail pharmacies for diarrhoea and to analyze the implications of such practices for the diarrhoea problem. Specifically, it sought to document what retail pharmacies prescribe for watery and bloody diarrhoea of children.

Methods

The study used a combination of survey (open survey and confederates survey) and direct observation to generate data. The open survey generated data on socio-demographic characteristics of operators; their educational and professional qualifications; their knowledge of diarrhoea and ORT; and their self-reported prescription for diarrhoea. The confederates survey obtained data (in disguise) on actual prescriptions for diarrhoea. Confederates posed as parents with children suffering from diarrhoea whose description fitted either watery or bloody diarrhoea. The idea of using data from an open and a confederates survey was to enable comparison to be made between what pharmacists say they prescribe and what they actually prescribe. Field assistants were sent to interview all operators of retail pharmacies and patent medicine shops in Maiduguri; Gamboru; Konduga; Gubio; Dikwa; Benisheik; Damboa and Monguno, all in Borno State, Nigeria. When this survey was completed, confederates were sent to the same pharmacies and patent medicine shops to present with children with either acute watery or acute bloody diarrhoea. They were instructed to buy all that were prescribed. Thus there were two sets of data for each pharmacy or patent medicine shop. The data reported here is only a part of a much larger data.

Results

Table 19.1
Type of licence and prescription given for watery diarrhoea

Type of licence	Prescription given for watery diarrhoea			
	Drugs only	Drugs & ORT	only ORT	Total
Pharmaceutical chemist	50	7	-	57
Patent medicine shop	74	-	2	76
Total	124	7	2	133

Table 19.1, shows that in a majority of pharmacies, children who were presented with watery diarrhoea, were prescribed "only drugs". In this there was no significant difference between the pharmaceutical chemists (87.7%) and the patent medicine shops (97.3%). Table 19.1, gives a lambda value of zero (with type of licence as independent variable). This indicates that knowing the licence under which a retail pharmacy is established, does not in any way, help us to predict what it is likely to prescribe for watery diarrhoea. The logical expectation is for facilities operated under pharmaceutical licence to prescribe more rationally than patent medicine shops, by giving the children ORT instead of non-rehydration medications. But we find that the seven pharmacies that prescribed ORT, prescribed it along with non-rehydration medications. In contrast, the two patent shops that prescribed ORT, gave it alone, without any drugs. This is the recommended treatment for watery diarrhoea. Drugs, whether antibiotic, antimicrobial or antimotility, are not recommended for watery diarrhoea.

Table 19.2

Type of licence and drugs given for watery diarrhoea

Type of licence	Drugs given for watery diarrhoea				
	Antibiotics	Antibiotics & Anti-diarrhoea drugs	Antidiarrh. drugs only	Antidiarr antibiotic & other drugs	Total
Pharm. chemist	7	11	33	4	55
Patent medicine shop	19	14	36	1	70
Total	26	25	69	5	125

Table 19.2, gives a chi-square value of 3.47, which is not significant at any level (given the 3 degrees of freedom), and a lambda value of zero (with type of licence as the independent variable). The chi-square value indicates that there is no significant difference between pharmaceutical chemists and patent medicine shops in the drugs they prescribed for watery diarrhoea. The lambda value indicates that knowing the type of licence of a retail pharmacy, does not help in any way in predicting the type of drug likely to be prescribed for watery diarrhoea. This comes out clearly when we examine the data more closely. When we examine the cells, we find that for "antibiotics only", pharmaceutical chemists has 12.7% and patent medicine shops, 27%. For the combination of "antibiotics and antidiarrhoea drugs" there is an equal 20% for each category of licence that prescribed it. But for "antidiarrhoea drugs only" there is a difference, with 60% of pharmaceutical chemists as against 51.4% of patent medicine shops prescribing it. And for the combination of "antibiotics, antidiarrhoea and other drugs" we have a distribution of 7.2% for pharmaceutical chemists as against 1.4% for patent medicine shops. Thus although there are some differences between these percentage distributions, these differences are not significant, as shown by the chi-square statistic. Antidiarrhoea drugs were prescribed by the majority of both pharmaceutical chemists and patent medicine shops. These were mainly antimotility preparations, usually the kaolin-pectin combination. The antibiotics included metronidazole (flagyl), which was the most frequently prescribed; ampicillin; terramycin; and cotrimoxazole. Other antimicrobial agents such as cloxacillin, amoxycillin and guanamycin, were also prescribed.

Table 19.3, gives a lambda value of zero, indicating that knowledge of type of licence does not help us, in any way, to predict whether or not, a pharmacy will prescribe ORT and the type of ORT likely to be prescribed. There was no significant difference between pharmaceutical chemists and patent medicine shops in the prescription of ORT.

Table 19.3
Type of licence and prescription of ORT

Type of licence	ORT Prescribed				
	ORS sachet	SSS recomm. but not taught	SSS recomm. and taught	ORT not prescribed	Total
Pharm. chemists	5	1	1	50	57
Patent medicine shops	1	-	1	75	77
Total	6	1	2	125	134

Discussion of the results

One of the important findings of this study is the widespread irrational use of drugs in the treatment of watery diarrhoea. First, there is the widespread use of kaolin and pectin combinations and other antimotility preparations for childhood diarrhoea. It has been demonstrated conclusively, that these antimotility preparations are not only useless for the application, but could in fact be dangerous and their use a threat to the lives of the children (Tomson, 1990; WHO, 1990). Tomson (1990) has suggested that kaolin and pectin preparations, tetracyclin and other antimotilitics in formulations for small children be banned because of their danger. I strongly advocate that the Federal Government of Nigeria adopt this sensible suggestion. The use of these drugs for childhood diarrhoea is not only dangerous, it also represents misallocation and waste of scarce resources.

The abuse of antibiotics for diarrhoea is another aspect of this irrational use of drugs for diarrhoea. Such abuse of antibiotics for watery diarrhoea and in particular by means of prescriptions from retail pharmacies, have been reported from other parts of the developing world. For example, Tomson and Sterky (1986) have reported such abuse from Bangladesh, Sri Lanka and Yemen; and Thamlikitkul (1988) from Thailand.

The abuse of antibiotics in the treatment of watery diarrhoea, has far-reaching negative consequences for diarrhoea control programmes. The most obvious is the possibility of the emergence of microbial strains that are resistant to existing chemotherapeutics, a development that can render useless treatment regimens for many debilitating diseases. In fact, the Pharmaceutical Society of Nigeria (PSN) has reported that most of the causative micro-organisms for diarrhoea in the country, are either already resistant, or are developing resistance to existing antibiotics.

The Federal Government must therefore start to devise ways of controlling access to antibiotics. We are aware that this is going to be very difficult. But it is a problem that health development in the country must confront now before it is too late.

Another implication of the irrational use of non-rehydration medications for watery diarrhoea is that parents are being made to spend hard-earned incomes that are desperately needed to finance other pressing needs, such as nutrition, on drugs that are not indicated, that are useless for the application, and that may actually be dangerous. In addition, attention is focused on drugs and not ORT. This neglect of ORT could increase case fatality rates for watery diarrhoea.

But what are the reasons for this unscientific prescribing on the part of pharmacies?It could be attributed partly to lack of knowledge and information. This could be corrected by a programme of education. A more important reason in the Nigerian context is the profit motive of retail pharmacies. More profit could be made by prescribing expensive antibiotics, antimicrobial and antidiarrhoeal drugs than selling cheap ORS sachet or teaching parents, for no fee, to prepare and use salt sugar solution at home. Attempts to improve prescribing must recognize the legitimacy of the profit motive on the part of businesses like pharmacy and address it with specific strategies.

It has also been reported that pharmacies do not prescribe ORT because mothers are not satisfied with it. It is reported that mothers expect ORS to stop diarrhoea as a "medicine", and complain when it does not (Bentley, 1988; Chowdhury, et al., 1991). A similar point was made by the pharmacists during the focus group discussions in this study. The pharmacists pointed out that mothers expect ORS to be a cure. They expect to be given a cure when they come to the pharmacy. A pharmacy that refuses to prescribe cures will be avoided for those that do, thus making such pharmacies miss out on the money to be made. This expectation on the part of the mothers could be corrected by education.

Another point implicit in this study is the widespread use of retail pharmacies as outpatient clinics. It would seem to me that the Federal Government must now take a second look at the legal position regarding outpatient clinical practice by retail pharmacies. The legislation now needs to be changed to recognize the reality. This call appears logical when one compares the pharmacist with a university degree, with the village health worker, who is to be trained under the PHC scheme, to be in charge of village health centres.

Another dimension is the double illegality in which patent medicine shops are engaged. They prescribe and handle poisons and treat patients, contrary to their licence. The operators are not trained in any formal way and their practices are therefore very dangerous. Government must now begin the process of phasing out this category of licence altogether.

References

Bentley, M.E. (1988). 'The household management of childhood diarrhoea in rural India'. *Social Science and Medicine*, 27, 75-86.

Chowdhury, A. *et al.*; (1991). Cereal-based ORT. Pros and Cons. Dialogue on Diarrhoea, 44, March.

Dressler, W.W. (1982). Hypertension and culture change. Acculturation and disease in the West Indies. South Salem, New York Redgrave.

Ferguson, A.E. (1981). 'Commercial pharmaceutical medicine and medicalization: a case study from EL Salvador'. *Culture, Medicine and Psychiatry*, 5, 105-134.

Haak, H. (1988). 'Pharmaceuticals in two Brazilian villages: Lay practices and perception'. *Social Science and Medicine*, 27, (12) 1415-1427.

Igun, U.A. (1982). 'Child-feeding habits in a situation of social change: the case of Maiduguri, Nigeria'. *Social Science and Medicine*, 16, 769-781.

Igun, U.A. (1987). 'Why we seek treatment here: retail pharmacy and clinical practice in Maiduguri, Nigeria'. *Social Science and Medicine*, 24, 8, 689-695.

Logan, K. (1983). 'The role of pharmacists and over the counter medications in the health care system of a Mexican city'. *Medical Anthropology*, 7, 68-89.

Mabadeje, A.F.B. (1974). The epidemiology of drug usage in metropolitan Lagos. In Bagshawe, *et al.* (ed): The Use and Abuse of Drugs and Chemicals in Tropical Africa. Nairobi. East African Literature Bureau.

Merson, M.H. (1988). World overview. In Prather (ed.): *Proceedings of the Third International Conference on ORT,* 23-31.

Mitchell, F.M. (1983). 'Popular medical concepts in Jamaica and their impact on drug use'. *Western Journal of Medicine*, 139 841-847.

Nichter, M. (1983). 'Paying for what ails you: socio-cultural issues influencing the ways and means of therapy payment in South India'. *Social Science and Medicine*, 17, 957-965.

Price, L.J. (1989). 'In the Shadow of biomedicine: Self-medication in two Ecuadorian Pharmacies'. *Social Science and Medicine*, 28, 9, 1015.

Sussman, L.K. (1981). 'Unity in diversity in a polyethnic society: the maintenance of medical pluralism in Mauritius'. *Social Science and Medicine*, 15B, 247-260,

Thamlikitkul, V. (1988). 'Antibiotic dispensing by drug store personnel in Bangkok, Thailand'. *Journal of Antimicrobial Chemotherapy*, 21, 125-131.

Tomson, G. and Sterky, G. (1986). 'Self-prescribing by way of pharmacies in three Asian developing countries'. *The Lancet*, 2, 620-622.

Tomson, G. (1990). Drug utilization studies in Sri Lanka: Towards an understanding of medicines in society. Stockholm, Sweden, IHCAR.

van der.Geest S. (1982). 'The illegal distribution of western medicines in developing countries: Pharmacies, drug pedlars, injection doctors and others. A bibliographic exploration'. *Medical Anthropology*, 6, (4) 197-219.

WHO: (1990). The rational use of drugs in the management of acute diarrhoea in children. Geneva, WHO.

Wolffers, I. (1987). Drug information and sale practices in some pharmacies of Colombo, Sri Lanka. *Social Science and Medicine*, 25, 319-321.

20 Primary health care and consumer behaviour in Kingston, Jamaica

Elizabeth M. Thomas-Hope

Summary

Analysis of the Jamaica health service is usually undertaken from a perspective which pays little attention to its sustainability in the long run. Yet, at both official and individual levels, the pressures upon financial resources are increasing.

This paper examines the nature of health care behaviour in a spontaneous settlement of the capital, Kingston. In terms of the demographic and economic characteristics of the community, it is typical of other poor urban communities in Jamaica, but in terms of access to primary health clinics, it is located in an area of the city where public provisions are at their best within the national context.

The pattern of health care behaviour among this urban population demonstrates considerable over-emphasis on the use of the available clinics, with heavy resource to them for illnesses which would have been more effectively dealt with by environmental and preventive measure. Furthermore, the use of prophylactics derived from local flora was a traditional practice, now largely lost by the urban populations. As a consequence, basic health treatments are purchased at very high relative cost to the individual, while serious pressures are placed upon national funds for sustaining the required or expected levels of health care provision in a situation of diminishing resources.

The paper argues that a critical element in the process of structural readjustment of the health sector should include the evaluation of consumer expectations and practices with regard to the utilization of the service.

Introduction

At the heart of the current crisis in the Jamaican health service is the increasing divergence of popular practices and expectations from the economic ability of the country to sustain them. While traditional approaches to health care have been eroded over the past half century, especially in urban areas, many of the traditional expectations of the curative properties of all medicine and the powerful, even prophetic, nature of medical practitioners remain as latent beliefs which condition health care behaviour. This situation has the potential of leading to a widening gulf between consumer expectations and practice on the one hand and the resources of both the national budget and private individual on the other.

The issue of health care behaviour at the level of the consumer is raised in this paper in order to assess its appropriateness for the system of primary care current in Jamaica. This is a system which is developed on the basis of western models of allopathic health care and delivered through a network of government clinics, private general and specialist practices and one urban clinic, Foundation International Self Help (FISH), operating in the voluntary sector as a Non-Governmental Organization.

The health sector in Jamaican context

The problems encountered in the provision of health care in Jamaica have to be seen within the wider context of structural adjustment necessitated by the current implications of the national debt and the conditions of the international creditors. Periods of expansion in the sector, accompanied by increasing expectations, have been followed by periods of readjustment of budgetary restrictions. At no time in the past has this process of readjustment been more painful than at the present.

Since 1982, the level of real expenditure on health services declined sharply over the previous five-year period. According to a UNICEF report, real expenditure in Jamaica on services such as education, health and social security fell from Ja$662 million in 1981-82 to Ja$372 million in 1985-86, a reduction of 44% over that of five year period. The relative decline was due largely to the increasing cost of drugs and medical supplies which were imported and rising dramatically in real costs because of the major devaluations of the Jamaican dollar which had occurred over the same period (for example, a 50% reduction in value against the US dollar took place in late 1991 in just one devaluation).

The UNICEF study also showed that the combined effect of the rising cost of living and decreased health care was that both mortality from curable diseases and malnutrition was on the increase. In Jamaica the percentage of malnourished children under four years of age rose from an estimated 38% in 1978 to 41% in 1985. The percentage of children under five admitted to the Bustamante Children's Hospital suffering from malnutrition and/or gastroenteritis rose from 2.7% of all admissions in 1980 to 8.4% in 1985. Similarly, the percentage of pregnant women screened at ante-natal clinics who were deemed anaemic rose from 23% in 1981 to 43% in 1985. Moreover, the infant mortality rate increased from 16 per 1,000 in 1980 to 18 per 1,000 in 1987 (Musgrave cited in Deere, 1990, p. 60).

Awareness that the demands on the national health service are related to levels of education, employment and environmental conditions (particularly as they affect living conditions) have been incorporated into ideas relating to health planning (See Cumper, 1972, 101-106; and Smith, 1989, 75-88). While these factors are critical ones in the advancement of a workable health system, they tend to provide a diversion away from the immediate issue in health care. First, improvements in standards of education, employment and living conditions are also dependent on the state of the economy. Second, they are all subject to the same loan restrictions as that of health because of their non-productive nature. Third, like health, they are associated with the import rather than export of products and so suffer most through currency devaluations and the indirect effect of recessions in the countries upon which they traditionally turn for assistance. To rely on the fundamental structural adjustments in the economy which would ultimately facilitate major changes in employment, education and living conditions in keeping with Western models to revolutionize health, is clearly to be stuck in a pragmatic cul-de-sac even though conceptually it may seem to offer a break-through.

Each time the crisis in health has been keenly felt in Jamaica, adjustments have followed a reactive path of accommodation, rather than forging a path towards the development of more creative or radical change. In the 1970s Jamaica chose to facilitate Primary Health Care Development through international loan financing, which in itself demonstrated a commitment to the objective of providing a comprehensive system of primary health care. Programmes contained some interesting developments involving the notion of Community Participation and Self Help. A Nurse Practitioner Training Scheme and Community Health Aid projects were initiated, and priorities were specified in maternal and child health.

These ideas never had the opportunity of being fully developed due to lack of funding (nor were they inherently radical in terms of content). By the late 1970s the focus had shifted back towards the search for international aid to maintain the status quo. A number of specific projects were funded and implemented to facilitate this form of development.

Projects in the Kingston Metropolitan Area (KMA) were financed by the Norwegian Government, while in the County of Cornwall, in western Jamaica, another scheme was funded to the tune of seven million dollars by the World Bank and the Government of Jamaica. This project provided for the construction and equipping of 56 primary health centres (Tulloch, 1986, 107). In the 1982-85 period a Health Management Improvement project was financed by the United States Agency for International Development (USAID).

However radical at times the approach to health may have appeared to be in the past, especially in the 1970s, the radicalism, insofar as it existed at all, was only at the political level. The approach has always been conservative at the conceptual level and the paradigms concerning health care and primary health care in particular have not significantly departed from current Western models. It is here suggested that a reorientation of emphasis to focus efforts on trying to understand the health behaviour of the majority of the population, and to alter the pattern of health care delivery accordingly, would be a valuable approach to the situation.

The case study - settlements in the Hope Valley

The settlements selected for the study on which the paper reports are typical of other poor urban communities, as the characteristics of the sample shows, but in terms of access to primary health care they are located in one of the areas of the city best served by health facilities (Bailey and Phillips, 1990). Therefore, pattern of health care provision is not here to be confused with the lack of clinics, but instead, on the health care behaviour given the provision at its best within the Jamaican context.

In the decade of the 1960s, Jamaica's ten largest settlements absorbed almost 90% of the island's population growth. Kingston, Jamaica's primate city, became the outstanding target, absorbing one half of the total amount. By the 1980s the KMA had experienced a population increase of 200,000 over the 1970 total and was the location of one third of the island's population (Clarke, 1983).

Like all other river valleys and gullies running through the KMA, the Hope Valley is the location of settlements developed since the 1960s. These represented a second phase of squatter growth, the first being between the marsh land along the shore and the main road into the city from the West. This rapid population increase had a profound impact on the urban system, placing a severe strain upon its employment, housing capacity and services.

The settlements of the Hope River Valley grew as lots were leased from the government for building purposes in the early 1960s. Since then, they have grown by accretion up the steep hillsides and away from the main roads and service provisions, or else by infilling with plots of land becoming let and sublet.

The field data discussed in this paper were based on sample survey involving 500 households. The study area encompassed two of the four settlements in the gully - the one, Tavern, on the west side of the gully, the other on the east - Kintyre (Fig. 20.1).

Despite a considerable range in the condition of the houses in any one of the districts, in general terms the older and most upgraded and substantial houses were located closest to the main road which formed the western perimeter of the area. The closer to the river bed itself and the farther south and east, away from the main transportation routes, the more recent and the poorer the condition of the dwellings.

Characteristics of the communities

One observable feature was the youthful nature of the population with most heads of households in their 40s. Although the average number of children was only 2-3, a great range existed and 6.4% of the households of lower Tavern recorded more than 7 children.

The average size of household was 5. The majority of households were female headed, the most extreme example being in lower Tavern, where 80% of the heads were female.

Education and employment levels showed little variation throughout the area. Few household heads had achieved completion of a secondary education and obtained a certificate. Many had not completed primary school and the few who had gone to a secondary school had not finished their course of study.

Formal employment levels throughout the communities were low with unemployment rates ranging from levels 21.2 to 41.9% in upper

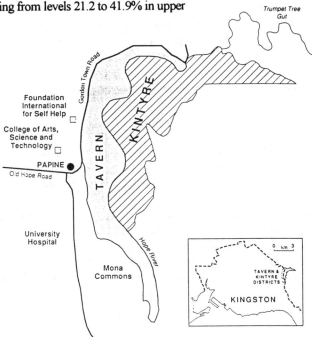

Figure 20.1   Tavern and Kintyre districts, Kingston, Jamaica

and lower Tavern respectively. Of those in work, over half were in full-time occupation, with domestic work being by far the most prevalent (12.4%). Some of those declaring to be unemployed were, in fact, involved in some form of informal commercial activity, but this was difficult to monitor as much of it was intermittent. Also noted in other work in urban areas (for example, Eyre, 1984), people invariably disregarded informal activity as employment and reported themselves to be unemployed.

Housing quality reflected very wide discrepancies. In terms of tenure, owner occupation was the dominant form, except in the case of upper Tavern where they were more rented units (51.5%). The rented units were in many cases part of the same yard (compound) in which the owner also lived. The number of rooms within these dwellings were on average 2 or 3.

With respect to housing conditions, upper Tavern, which occupied the most favourable location at the base of the valley and up the western slopes to the main road, was the best established section in the valley. Some 60% of the dwellings in this area were constructed of concrete and 80% of the households had their own water supply. Similarly, households in this district were best equipped with amenities, such as kitchens inside the house (78.9%) and inside toilets (63.6%).

In contrast, Kintyre, located on the east side of the valley, was farthest from the main service provisions and transport and appeared to be the worst off in nearly all respects. Only 62.2% of the households had water from mains supplies, and only 43.6% had inside toilets. In terms of material conditions, the households in this district were generally the poorest and least equipped in terms of household items and furniture.

Primary health care provisions in the locality

These settlements were in close proximity to the University hospital, a government clinic at Gordon Town some 8 km away, a number of private practitioners within a 4.8 km radius, and in the immediate catchment of the Foundation International Self Help (FISH) clinic.

The hospital clinics offered services and medication at nominal cost but attendance involved very long waiting times. The government clinic at Gordon Town made no charge for medical consultation and basic treatment, but most medications prescribed had to be purchased from private pharmacies. The FISH clinic, established in 1985 by voluntary initiatives, was partially supported, as a non-governmental organization, by grants from overseas (chiefly Canada), by charitable donations and the (subsidized) payments made by the patients. The facilities at FISH cost more than at the hospital (though they were still nominal).

People in the Hope River communities rarely ever went to private practitioners because of the easy access to much cheaper services in the vicinity. Decisions concerning the choice of the clinics were usually made on practical grounds. These were chiefly distance of home to the clinics and the evaluation of the importance of waiting time versus cost.

There were also known areas of specialization at the two centres and patients were highly discriminating in their use of the clinics on the basis of this knowledge. Those patients requiring ante-natal and family planning services chiefly went to hospital clinics, while for optical and dental treatment, they went to FISH. There were also attempts to provide diabetes and high blood pressure education at the FISH centre.

One implication of the waiting time versus cost basis of decision-making in the use of clinics, was that at times of additional economic hardship cost became by far the most important determining factor - even exceeding the criterion of known specialization. The services at FISH became severely underused, thus potentially posing a threat to the continued viability of the clinic itself. With the diversion of patients to the cheaper government provisions, these in turn became commensurately over-crowded and resources over-burdened. As a result, the long waiting times which in the first place had deterred people when they could afford the alternative became even longer as more people were faced with no feasible alternative. The existence of the government clinics as acceptable means of health care delivery could also become threatened in times of economic difficulty. Since these were the very same times of structural readjustment when the national budget was also over-stretched, the entire system of health care entered a phase of crisis.

Health care behaviour

Despite some variation in the socio-economic circumstances of the members of the Hope Valley communities, this was not of major significance in terms of health care behaviour. Neither reason for visiting doctors nor frequency of visits varied significantly, though expenditure on medication and the type of pharmaceutical preparations purchased did bear some relationship to income levels.

Adult health

The main reason for the last visit made to a doctor by adults in the area, was sickness due to some form of gastric disorder (31.1%). The second most prominent reason was for conditions relating to high blood pressure (15.6%). Well over half the adult population (57.5%) had been to the doctor within the previous twelve weeks and an additional 25% within the previous two weeks. Thus, more than three quarters of the adult population had visited a health clinic within three months.

In terms of the pattern of visiting a clinic at the actual time of feeling unwell, there was a high incidence of early visits, many within the same day. Overall, taking both Tavern and Kintyre together, some 25% of the sample population had visited a clinic within the previous two weeks, 58% within two and twelve weeks, 15.5% within three and twelve months; only 1.5% rarely or never used the clinics.

Furthermore, of the reasons for the last visit to a doctor, 15.5% had been for a check-up.

Many people would have preferred to have gone to a doctor even sooner than they had but were deterred from doing so because of the lack of money. This was the case in more than half (52.8%) the number of situations of delay. This would certainly have included some persons who ought to have received prompt medical attention. Other cases of inaccessibility included 2.7% of those who wanted to get to a doctor sooner but were delayed because they were too ill (or immobile) to get there and a further 2.7% because they were unable (or felt unable) to go alone and had non-one available to accompany them. The over-use of clinics by some and the under-use by others raise issues of major concern in this context of primary health care.

The level of satisfaction with the services received at the clinics was generally high. Most people were very satisfied with both the treatment they received from the doctor and the medicine or advice they were given. About a third of the population were fairly satisfied and only a very small minority (some 2.2%) were not at all satisfied.

The mere fact of being seen by a doctor was in itself regarded as a reason to be satisfied. People rarely applied remedies themselves without also seeking the advice of a doctor, unless they were unable to afford this reassurance. Certainly, the amount spent on health care in these communities reflected the distribution of wealth within the community itself. In the economically better-off areas, 53.7% of the population had spent over (Jamaican)$35 in the previous three months on fees to clinics and 32.6% on medication. In the poorer areas, 18.8% had spent over $35 on doctors and 22.9% on medicines in the same period. As long as people were able to see a doctor, there appeared to be no apparent relationship between the level of satisfaction with the type of treatment received and the amount spent.

Medicines taken

A further aspect of concern in the nature of health care behaviour in the urban communities was the high level of expenditure on expensive preparations when cheap, easily accessible alternatives would have been appropriate. In particular, there was a relatively high level of expenditure on tonics and laxatives. In one of the areas in the sample some 40% of the households had purchased tonics as a means of health care, in the same areas 14% of households had purchased laxatives. Though the overall figure for the reliance on tonics and laxatives was high throughout the communities, it was in the poorest areas that this was greatest. In some cases these were taken as a substitute for going to the clinic but in many cases were purchased in addition to seeing a doctor.

Child health

Morbidity among children was due primarily to dietary factors and sanitation, with illnesses relating to gastric disorders and malnutrition. It is significant to note that in the poorest area in the study, some 61% of the households indicated that their children were receiving sufficient food and 46% felt that it was the right kind of food for children's nutritional needs. Yet in the economically better-off areas of the settlement fewer (49%) were satisfied that their children had enough food. Perceptions and understanding of nutritional requirements of children were clearly an area which needed attention, though the high cost of food relative to household budgets, especially in urban areas, would defeat most objectives of nutritional programmes. The problem is a difficult one to tackle, but in any case, much of the morbidity among children required the type of input which would be more effective at the preventive stage rather than relying on the ameliorative effects of allopathic medicine.

Conclusion

Reliance on formal provisions of primary health care have been accompanied by an over-emphasis on the use of such services and the high expectation of provision of curative medicine. This places considerable pressure upon resources for sustaining the required or expected level of provision in the context of diminishing resources. There is a commensurate lack of resources which could be used for treatment of the seriously ill, the least socially accessible groups, and on preventive aspects of the service. At both official and individual levels, the pressures upon financial resources are increasing.

First, the attempt to create a comprehensive national system of allopathic medicine cannot be sustained without continuing and increasing dependence on external aid. Second, consumer behaviour needs to be carefully examined within the context of existing national and personal budgetary constraints. While there is a demand for increased national health services, expectations are based upon a concept of health which developed on the basis of traditional practice and understanding and which are being transferred to the modern system. At the same time, the individual responsibility taken for health at the level of the individual and family has been eroded with modern, especially urban living. Along with this has occurred the growing lack of responsibility and involvement on the part of the community for the health of the community.

The pattern of health behaviour which has developed demonstrates a deeply entrenched dependence on the government by the people at the one level, and on the international community by the government at the official level. From the point of view of the people, the objective is to obtain more medicine at lower cost. The response of government continues to attempt to increase Western produced drugs and technology to meet demand. Under current economic constraints necessitating structural readjustment in all aspects of Caribbean welfare provision, the health service faces a major crisis.

Analysis of the health service is usually undertaken from a perspective based on models not only alien to, but inconsistent with, the sustainability of the service in the long term. In the present context, the historically developed, traditional approaches to health and well-being and the form and use of therapy was well tuned to the social, economic and environmental systems which pertained. In the second half of the twentieth century, the model of health care and the accompanying expectations and practices associated with it have diverged more and more from the economic basis whereby it could be sustained. The commensurate loss of alternatives which were or could be consistent with local conditions and economic levels have left societies and the services they expect, stranded as the economic tide of temporary prosperity and international assistance has receded.

It would appear that a critical element in the process of readjustment should be the evaluation of existing practices and attitudes with regard to the utilization of the health service. The objective would be to reduce the current heavy reliance on an assumption that high quality, comprehensive and affordable primary health care can be provided in a context such as that of Jamaica in the decade towards the 21st century. The issue of developing a plural model of health care requires further research.

References

Bailey, W. and Phillips, D.R. (1990). Spatial patterns of use of health services in the Kingston Metropolitan Area, Jamaica. *Social Science and Medicine.* 30, (1) 1-12.

Bannerman, R.H., Burton, J. and Che'en, W.C. (eds.), (1983). *Traditional Medicine and Health Care Coverage.* Geneva, WHO.

Boyd, D. (1988). The impact of adjustment policies on vulnerable groups: the case of Jamaica 1973-1985. In Giovanni Cornea, R. Jolly and F. Stewart (eds.) Adjustment with a Human Face (New York, Clarendon Press/UNICEF. Vol. II, 130-45.

Clarke, C.G. (1983). Dependency and marginality in Kingston, Jamaica. Geography. 82, (5) 227-35.

Cumper, G. (1972). Survey of Social Legislation in Jamaica (Mon. Jamaica, Institute of Social and Economic Research.

Deere, C. D. (1990). In the shadows of the Sun: Caribbean Development Alternatives and U.S. Policy. Boulder, Westview Press.

Eyre, L.A. (1984). The internal dynamics of Jamaica's shanty towns. Caribbean Geography. 1, (4) 256-71.

LeFranc, E. 0. (1990). Health status and health services utilization in the English-speaking Caribbean. (Mona, Jamaica, Institute of Social and Economic Research.

Musgrave, P. (1987). The economic crisis and its impact on health and health care in Latin America and the Caribbean. *International Journal of Health Services.* 7 (3) 418-27.

Norton, A.. (1978). *Shanties and Skyscrapers: Growth and Structures of Modern Kingston.* Cave Hill, Barbados, Institute of Social and Economic Research, Working Paper No. 13.

Phillips, D.R. (1990). *Health and Health Care in the Third World.* London, Longmans.

Smith, M.G. (1989). *Poverty in Jamaica,* Mona, Jamaica, Institute of Social and Economic Research.

Tulloch, E.E., *Planning the Health Sector: The Jamaica Perspective.* Unpublished Ph.D. thesis, University of Liverpool, 1986.

21 The population of mentally disadvantaged in Nigeria: Health and development programme

E. A. Emeke and T. W. Yoloye

Summary

The paper considered the fact that the actual population of the mentally disadvantaged in Nigeria needs to be known, so that its economic importance on the overall development of the country can be assessed. By projection, and using comparative assessment methods from Nigeria and other countries, the writers estimated the population of the mentally disadvantaged in Nigeria to be 1.77 million, and submit that this has grave consequences on the health programme and the general development of the nation.

The writers contend that at present, Nigeria does not have adequate health facilities and programmes for its mentally disadvantaged citizens. However, attempts at provision of facilities can be found based in the homes of the mentally disadvantaged, in educational institutions, hospitals and at governmental level.

The productivity of the mentally disadvantaged is very low, and to provide food, water, shelter, and other amenities to almost 2 million mentally disadvantaged in a depressed economy will have a tremendously negative effect on Nigeria's development. The paper concluded that the situation can however be made better and the mentally disadvantaged can contribute their own quota to the per-capita earnings of the nation. This could be achieved by making them productive through adequate training and provision of educative health programmes that have legislative backing. More researches and the use of therapeutic methods could help the mentally disadvantaged to learn and cope with some life situations. Urban designs should accommodate the mentally disadvantaged and the social integration strategies should be more humane and all embracing.

Introduction

Although reliable statistics of the mentally disadvantaged and mentally ill people in many developing countries of Africa and Asia are not available, a cursory observation from the street corners, health centres, mental homes, cheshire and other humanitarian homes indicate that the number is very high.

Mba (1986) reported that there were an estimated 857,007 children of the primary school age with behaviour disorder, 422,053 mentally disadvantaged and 182,749 with learning disability in Nigeria. Although there was no evidence about the procedure employed to arrive at these figures, however if one should observe the figures for the children of primary school age alone, then the figure for all groups of people on population of the country will be very high.

There are various ways in which the number of a smaller group e.g. mentally disadvantaged people could be known in any population. This could include the physical counting of the individual or a projection from a small sample to the total population.

In the 1991 census in Nigeria, the National Population Commission had the intention to have physical count of all individuals including the mentally disadvantaged and mentally ill. The mentally ill people were supposed to be counted at night. However due to some logistic problems like looking for 'mad people' at night the Commission decided to rely on projection.

It should also be noted, that there are differences between the mentally ill and mentally disadvantaged individuals. While the mentally ill individuals are those with mental or behaviour disorders, the mentally disadvantaged are those with slow mental or cognitive development. The mentally disadvantaged can be classified into two major classes, namely:

1. the organically pathological mentally disadvantaged whose IQ ranges between 0-70, and
2. the non-organically familiar mentally disadvantaged with IQ ranging between 50-70.

Whether, the Nigerian National Population Commission, takes this distinction into consideration or not we are not sure. It may even be of no interest to the Commission to think about the mentally disadvantaged people as those whose population needs to be known. However, it is our contention that through the adequate knowledge of the number of the disadvantaged , adequate planning and provision of health programmes can be done while the effect on the general development of the nation will be known.

Other problems could be lack of experts in the area of mentally disadvantaged who could help in classifying this group of people.

In as much as we are not pre-empting the outcome of the population count, we know that there are always conflicting reports among health practitioners on how to classify mentally disadvantaged people, and this could affect the outcome of any projection.

Over the years many workers in the area of mental handicap and mental health have focused on the issue of Intelligence Quotient (IQ) in classifying people as either normal or mentally disadvantaged. However, it is now known that the score of an individual on most of the measures and instruments on intelligence quotient could change most especially between the infancy and early childhood. Studies like those of Haunt (1971) and Lewis (1976) have pointed to this.

Also the individual's environment and experiences in life could lead to mis-labelling and classification of an individual as having low IQ For example, a Nigerian child who could not recognise some of the items in Wechlers Intelligence Scale for Children (WISC), Bayley Scale of Infant Development, McCarthy Scales of Children Abilities and many more 'Western' standardised tests that are totally irrelevant to the child's background could not be said to have a low IQ The child could recognise such items at a later year once he has been exposed to such experiences.

Again, if a Nigerian child could not read at the age of six years, such a child could not also be classified as having low IQ because it is possible he could be able to read at a later stage in life.

Many Africans are born into predominantly illiterate homes. A World Bank Report (1988) put the highest percentage of literate adults as 82.8% for Mauritius and the least as 11.6% for Somalia. For Nigeria the percentage is 42.4. Lack of literate adults to stimulate and act as role models for the African child and indeed Nigerian child born into less privileged and illiterate homes would not facilitate their walking, talking, reading etc. early in life and not necessarily that they have low IQ

We should not therefore employ IQ alone for the classification of the mentally disadvantaged, rather we should incorporate social, psychological, psychomotor, moti-vational factors, experiences as well as cultural background into the classification framework.

Some questions that readily come to the mind at this juncture include how many mentally disadvantaged people are in Nigeria? What are the health programmes and treatments that are available to the disadvantaged? What are the effects of the number of the mentally disadvantaged on the health programmes and the development of the Nation?

Determining the number of mentally disadvantaged in a population

Experts in the area of demography and population know that projection could be used to determine population from a subset or sample. Using projection to determine the number of mentally disadvantaged in a population therefore may not be too difficult and out of place.

Difficulties only usually arise in determining the characteristics of the sample - in this case the mentally disadvantaged. This is where an expert in the area of mental health will be relevant in the identification of the sample. Inability to do this often leads to mislabelling of people. For example, homeless people, dirty mechanic and automobile workers who are neither ill or retarded could be classified thus by non experts in the area of mental health.

In order to determine the number of mentally disadvantaged in a population therefore, could be:

(a) The selection of the sample area within a population. This could be by random cluster sampling or random stratified sampling in order to have a wider sample or geographical spread and easy generalisation.
(b) Expert should identify the mentally disadvantaged.
(c) There should be physical counting of the mentally disadvantaged in the sampled areas.
(d) The number of the disadvantaged in the sampled area could be used to project the number in a population.
(e) Projection from other studies

There are many studies that have examined the number of mentally disadvantaged in populations all over the world and the percentage estimate ranged from 0.6% to 3.5%. This differential estimate may be due to the location of the study, the age of the sample used and the test employed to identify the mentally disadvantaged.

The result of some of the studies are presented in Table 21.1.

Table 21.1

Percentage estimate of mentally disadvantaged from samples

Researcher	Location	Sample	Test employed	% Estimate
Akesson	Sweden	All diversified ages	Stanford Binet	1.75
Birch et al. (1970)	Scotland	8-10 years	Moray test	2.74
Merces (1973)	California	Diversified ages	Stanford Binet L.M. & Kuhlaman Binet	2.14
Reschly and Jipson (1976)	Arizona	1st 3rd 5th and 7th graders	WISC-R	3.53
Hagberg et al (1981)	Sweden	8-12 Terman	Swedish WISC & Terman Mernu	0.67
Adima (1989)	Nigeria	All diversified ages	Standford Binet and Physical count	2.0

As previously mentioned the differential percentage estimate of the mentally disadvantaged could be due to a number of factors like location, age of sample etc. Also it could reopen the debate about whether it is usually 1% or 3% of any population that are mentally disadvantaged.

Our contention is that sample and test administered should be related to the population and the cultural experiences of the sample. Also an estimate could be derived from all the six previous studies mentioned. Thus the number of researchers $n = 6$, the mean $X = 2.13$ and even the standard deviation is 0.96.

The mean score shows that there are 2.13% of the population from any of the nations sampled that are mentally disadvantaged. The assumption that 1% or 3% of any population is mentally disadvantaged may be baseless. After an extensive review of some prevalent studies, Zigler and Hodapp findings (1986) indicated that 2% to 2.5% of most population are mentally disadvantaged. Our findings of 2.13% support this view.

However, using Zigler and Hodapp findings (1986) and our own estimate of about 2%, then the projected estimate of the mentally disadvantaged people in Nigeria with a population of 88.5 million in accordance with the announced census figure of March, 1992 will be 1.77m or almost 2 million people. The problem therefore arises: how do we provide health programmes for the almost two million people? Are there enough health facilities and programmes in Nigeria?

Health programmes and treatment for the mentally disadvantaged In Nigeria

Many attempts and suggestions have been made in Nigeria to provide health facilities and treatment to the mentally disadvantaged. These attempts fall under four major categories namely:
1. The individual homes,
2. Educational institutions,
3. Hospitals and
4. Government level.

Home level

At the home level, the methods employed include:
   (a)   Taking the mentally disadvantaged to churches. Many Nigerians are religious and believe in the supernatural power of God to effect changes and healing in both themselves and their children, wards or relatives. It is against this background that one can understand the use of churches as healing/mediation centres for the mentally disadvantaged people at the home level.
   (b)   Taking the mentally disadvantaged to metaphysicists. This is still bordering to a larger extent on the religious tendency of Nigerians. Since not all are christians, others resort to metaphysicists who check the stars or crystal balls etc. to assess the cause of the problem and the possible way out.
   (c)   Taking the mentally disadvantaged to herbal homes. There are a good number of herbalists in Nigeria who use herbs and roots of plants to procure healing, and they claim they can heal any type of diseases and ailments.

Some if not all of the above-mentioned treatments at the home level have been said to be highly effective. But since the mechanism and scientific process are not easily known by us (the authors of this paper), we have scanty information. Also the percentage of those who preferred this method has not been investigated.

It must however be mentioned at this stage, that the attitude of many parents, other siblings and peer groups are negative and unfavourably disposed toward the mentally disadvantaged. There is social segregation and total lock up of the mentally disadvantaged in some homes. This negative attitude must be corrected.

Educational level

In the realm of education, attempt to provide health care and treatment for the mentally disadvantaged are in the area of researches, education and production of manpower.

In terms of research, many researchers from the universities, colleges of education and other research centres conduct and carry out researches in the area of mental handicapped and disadvantaged with a view to finding causes, possible physical and psychological treatments as well as suggestions to improve the health status of both the mentally disadvantaged and their parents/relatives.

The educational aspect is geared mainly towards education of others who are significant in the life of the mentally disadvantaged to accept the disadvantaged as individuals, improve their attitude towards them, teach them the very basic skills to practise with the disadvantaged as they grow up, and how to handle them generally. Counselling plays a major role in achievement of this education for the parents and guardians of the mentally disadvantaged.

In terms of manpower development, some of our universities and colleges of education are involved in the training of special education teachers and handlers who are later employed by state governments, charity homes and other social welfare organizations to teach and handle the mentally disadvantaged in the various areas. Though presently many schools and institutions produce special education teachers, it must however, be mentioned that the number of graduates produced from these institutions are inadequate. Adima (1988) even tried to prove that the special education and health workers who handle the mentally disadvantaged are those that have been rejected by other departments and fields. He also claimed that they are poorly prepared, due to lack of facilities in the various institutions.

Our finding on the cut-off points for admission into the University of Ibadan, College of Education, through the Joint Admission and Matriculation Board (JAMB) in Nigeria shows that the cut-off point for the Special Education Department is usually the lowest, followed by the Departments of Physical and Health Science Education, Adult Education, Arts Education, Educational Management and Guidance and Counselling. Thus a candidate with a score of 201 could be given admission to Special Education Department, while one with the score of 210 will not be able to get admission to the Department of

Educational Management or Guidance and Counselling because the mark is too low to the cut off point of 215.

The education and the production of health personnel for the mentally disadvantaged therefore needs to be improved upon in Nigeria.

Hospital level

Treatment and health provision at the hospital level focus on genetic treatment and use of exercises. In the case of genetic treatment, the use of drugs and vitamins to correct some defects in either the gene or physiological make up of the disadvantaged are often used. This method has been known to be highly effective with phenylketonuria (PKU).

The various organizations and mental health workers practise various exercise methods of treatment. This includes the Dorman Dalecto method. The method involves series of exercises and manipulations of limbs until correct neurological organization is achieved. For now, this method can be found in operation only in the Teaching Hospitals and a few other big centres. Another method, though not strictly located in a hospital setting is the use of music as embarked upon by Yoloye (1991).

Government level

The government is about the biggest single provider of the treatment and health provisions to the mentally disadvantaged.

Some of the methods employed at the government level include:

(i) Environmental treatment:- The age-long dichotomy between the geneticists and environmentalists were common occurrences among the mental health social workers in Nigeria. While studies like those of Okoye (1985) and Anagbogu (1986) were in favour of the environmental determinant and treatment or remediation, Nwaogu (1988) advocated genetic counselling. Yoloye (1991) on his own part recommended a combination of both the genetic and environmental approaches. The environmental treatment include slum and shanties reclaiming, urban and environmental planning, provision of side walks, social and recreations facilities including parks. Even the provision of special schools, or special classes within the regular school systems will be credited to the government in its efforts to provide health requirement of the mentally disadvantaged.

(ii) Establishment of rehabilitation centres, mental homes, mental hospitals and social welfare centres. These are scattered all over the country and are few in number. The government needs to improve its contribution in this regard.

(iii) Provision of funds is a third major area where government comes in. Government provides funds and equipment to the mentally ill, mentally disadvantaged and other handicaps either at the government or private rehabilitation centres, hospitals, mental homes etc. The funds and facilities are however, grossly inadequate. For example, the Federal College of Education (Special) Oyo, could not move to its permanent site up till now since its inception in 1977. This is over a period of fifteen years.

There are very few empirical studies on the efficacy of most of these programmes and methods of treatment in Nigeria. This could be a challenge, to us as experts in the area of health and development. Also, the cost-effectiveness of these programmes should be examined to see the impact on the economy and development of Nigeria.

Mentally disadvantaged population, health programme and development

The health of the mentally disadvantaged does not differ sharply, organically speaking, from the health of the normal population. The mentally disadvantaged does not more often than not, have other organic malformation aside of the central one - the brain - which is what in fact placed him in the category under question - the mentally disadvantaged. To this end, the mentally disadvantaged is not more prone to say malaria, or any such common diseases than any member of the "normal" population. The great difference, however, is that he is not able to cope with his treatment and medication as a "normal" person can. He thus needs a lot of care and attention when he becomes ill or indisposed. But when it is considered that even mental disadvantage is itself a health problem, then it will be appreciated that the health of the mentally disadvantaged to that extent differs from that of the "normal" population.

Mental disadvantage cannot be cured once it occurs. The objective of the "health" care for the group is not remission or recovery from the condition itself, but it is rather an attempt at making the mentally disadvantaged a bit functional in living, lessening the burdens of his parents, of those in charge of his care, and making him able to use programmes and services which will help him to attain an optimum level of functioning within the limitations of his own intellectual functioning. In that way, he can contribute his own little quota to the development of his society.

There is no doubt, that with our projected population of almost two million mentally disadvantaged individuals in Nigeria, in a SAP economy with poorly trained health workers, poor programmes and facilities, the effect on development will be tremendously negative. Little wonder therefore that many people roam the streets and more charitable organisations are joining the government to provide education and facilities to this group of people.

To provide food, water, shelter and other amenities to two million people who are mentally disadvantaged alone apart from other groups of handicaps, mentally ill and even the jobless in a developing nation as Nigeria will certainly affect overall development.

The productivity of the mentally disadvantaged is very low and they may not contribute positively to the per capita earnings of the nation. Rather they will depend on other individuals and the government thereby decreasing the per capita earnings of the country. This will always be the case in such countries, like Nigeria where the health programmes and treatments are very inadequate.

The mentally disadvantaged could be productive if adequate training and health facilities are provided. The mentally disadvantaged should not be locked up. We should be more humane towards them. The government should provide for them through adequate health programmes that have legislative backing. There should be more researches and therapeutic methods that could help the mentally disadvantaged to learn and cope with some situations.

It follows almost a cyclic sequence that if there is a well developed health programme and treatment methods the mentally disadvantaged will be able to develop coping mechanism, be productive and subsequently able to contribute to the development of the country.

The negative impact of poor health, education, social integration of the disadvantaged could be observed from the number of street beggars, poor sanitation and even urban slums in many cities in Nigeria. The effect is definitely negative on development.

As geographers, urban planners, educators, psychologists, social workers, government officials, our concern should be to know the number of mentally disadvantaged or any group and plan for them. Our urban designs should be one that should accommodate various groups, the education should be one that should make individuals to be more productive. The plans should provide for various groups in order to be able to develop and be more productive.

It is hoped that if this is done the seemingly high population of mentally disadvantaged will be provided for and the effect will not be drastic on the education, health and general development of the country.

Conclusion

There is no doubt that the number of the mentally disadvantaged in Nigeria is very high and the health programmes and treatments are not just poor but also include improper selection, training and funding of the programme and this has negative effects on the general development of Nigeria. However, it is our contention that through changes in the attitude of the parents, siblings, the general populace, positive changes in selection, training of personnel, adequate researches and health programmes, the poor situation could be changed to a positive one.

The mentally disadvantaged will be more productive and contribute their own quota to the development of the nation.

References

Adima, E.E. (1985). 'Present and future of special education in Nigeria'. *Journal of Education and Society,* University of Ife, 10.

Adima, E.E. (1988). 'Handicapping the handicap in Nigeria: Will the paradox end'? *Journal of Special Education* 4. 51-60.

Akesson, H.O. (1961). Epidemiology and genetics of mental deficiency in a Southern Swedish Population. Uppsala Almquist and Wiksell.

Anagbogu, M. A. (1986). 'Cognitive Limitation and its Improvement': *Nigerian Journal of Curriculum Studies* IV No. 1 56-66.

Birch, B.G. Richardson, S.A. Baird, D., Horobin, G. and Illsey, R. (1970). Mental Subnormality in the Community. A Clinical and Epidemiology Study, Balmimore, Williams and Vikins Co.

Hagberg, B., Hagbery, G., Lewearth, A., and Lindbery, U. (1981). 'Mild Mental Retardation in Swedish School Children. Prevalence'. *Acta Paediatrica Scandinavia*, 70, 1-8.

Hunt, J. M. (1971). Parent and Child Centres. Their basis in the behavioural and educational sciences. *American Journal of Orthopsychiatry*, 41, 13-38.

Lewis, M. (ed.) (1976). The origins of intelligence. New York: Plemun.

Mba, P.O. (1986). 'Manpower development diagnostic equipment materials and child clinics in Nigeria'. Paper presented at the National Workshop on Diagnostic Assessment, Kaduna.

Merler, J. (1973). Labelling the mentally disadvantaged. Berkeley, University of California Press.

Nwaogu, P. O. (1988). 'Genetic counselling. A case against birth defects and other social problems. *Journal of Special Education*. 4 pp. 61-67.

Okoye, N. N. (1985). 'Psychological stress associated with punishment and effect in learning'. In issues in *Teacher Education and Science Curriculum in Nigeria* No. 2, pp. 196-213.

Reachly, D. Jipson, F. (1976). 'Ethnicity, geographic locale, age, sex and urban rural residence in variables in the prevalence of mild disadvantaged'. *American Journal of Mental Deficiency.* 81, pp. 154-161.

World Bank Report (1988). Education in Sub-Sahara Africa.

Yoloye, T.W. (1991). 'Mental retardation and mental health. The Way Ahead'. Paper sent to International Conference on Mental Health the Way Ahead. Guys Thomas Hospital, London.

Zigler, E. and Robert, M. H. (1988). Understanding Mental Retardation. London, Cambridge Press.

22 Prevention of communicable diseases: Lessons from the expanded immunization programme in north-western Nigeria

Dora Shehu

Summary

In Nigeria, communicable diseases have consistently accounted for more than half of all illnesses affecting the population, the most vulnerable being the under-fives.

Immunization is a recognized prophylactic measure against the causative organism, but inadequate attention is given to the socio-ecological conditions which contribute to the susceptibility of the human body.

This chapter presents some selected cases of children for whom immunization has not worked partly on account of their material deprivation and partly on programme inadequacies. It calls for a rethinking of the programme drawing attention to the feasibility of approaching the problem of prevention from a radical community based angle.

Introduction

In Nigeria today communicable diseases continue to play an important role in the morbidity and mortality patterns of diseases. Of these, the childhood diseases - measles, whooping cough and tuberculosis are predominant, attacking thousands of children and causing needless deaths amongst the under fives. Even though the country has an immunization policy for children against measles, whooping cough, diphtheria, tetanus, tuberculosis and poliomyelitis, it has been estimated that about 200 out of every 1,000 babies die as a result of the preventable immunizable diseases (Chiwuzie, 1986). There has also been an expanded programme on immunization for nearly ten years but the trend does not appear to have changed in any appreciable manner (Fig. 22.1). There are several factors that may underlie this apparent inability substantially to reduce the level of infection amongst the population. Much of communicable diseases, in addition to their biomedical indices, also have an important socio-cultural dimension which is yet to be adequately addressed. Secondly, there are structural problems that relate directly to the economic development of the country and its effect on the health care system. There are also ecological factors which influence the disease organisms and the relationship which develop between man and the existing micro-organisms in a given area.

Research methodology

So far evaluative studies conducted on the status of immunization of children in the country have been based on surveys of uptake of immunization. (Alakija, 1980; Chiwuzie 1986; Erinosho, 1980). In this paper, use is made of case studies of real life situations of cases infected with communicable diseases for which immunization exist.

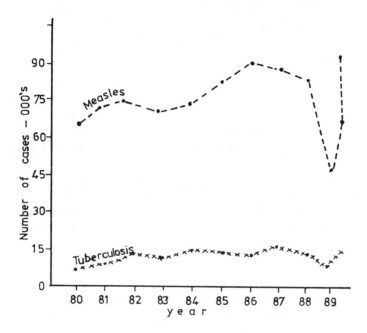

Figure 22.1   Trends in communicable diseases in Nigeria, 1980-89

These are taken from different areas of Sokoto State in North-western Nigeria. (Fig. 22.2) The studies throw light on such social factors and structural problems that beset the effort to control communicable diseases. Even though many cases could have been selected, for the sake of brevity only four are considered here. These are of *poliomyelitis, tuberculosis* and *measles*. All the cases reported at health centres in Sokoto and were followed to their respective homes.

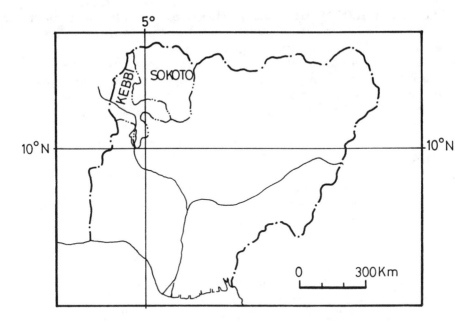

Figure 22.2   Map of Nigeria showing study area - Kebbi, Sokoto states

The cases describe a problematic situation and indicate the various experiences which people go through before they become infected. These experiences often reflect what generally occurs in the local environment and which could provide insight into the extent to which an immunization programme may or may not achieve its objectives.

In addition to the use of the case study a week was devoted to observing and studying the activities of the EPI programme and the paper considers some of the effects of the inadequate infrastructure on the success of the immunization programme.

Case no. 1

Farouk is a male child born in 1986 into a polygamous muslim family. He is the sixth child in a household of thirteen children. His father is a farmer, his mother, *mater auren (kulle),*[1] live in a self constructed compound house in Rinjim Sambo a suburb of Sokoto town. One of the original villages which has been engulfed by urban development and retains its rural features. It is a closely built up area with clay-walled compounds that contain individual mud-cum-cement houses. There is no provision of a proper sewage or drainage system, refuse is dumped on selected sites, most homes have wells, though a few are connected to pipe-borne supply.

259

Both parents have had koranic education and encourage and pay for their children to attend koranic classes, but none of them attends the formal system. His mother Rakiya has three other children two of who are older than Farouk.

When the fever first started, Rakiya thought it was an ordinary fever and she did nothing about it. Subsequently the boy got worse, and on being informed his father decided to take him to the hospital where he was admitted. The diagnosis was poliomyelitis. After what seemed a long time and with money spent, Farouk got better but he could no longer use his left leg.

Farouk had been born at home and his mother did not do much immunization. She took him to the clinic when he was about four months old where he was given some immunization, but she misplaced the card and did not return for any other. Nobody called to see her about it. The other children did not receive their full course either.

In any case she has been informed that the immunization is to prevent disease but then she believes that whatever Allah has prepared for one will always happen.

Case no. 2

Aiye is a girl, born in 1988, the first child of her mother Luba, who delivered her at home in her parents' house. After the fortieth day celebration, she went back to her husband's house with the baby. She never heard about immunizations and did not take the baby anywhere for that purpose. She lives in a village some 52km away from the nearest health centre.

Aiye was a healthy baby who did not have any serious illness that could not be handled in the village. When she was nearly three years old, her grandmother, Rabi took her to live with her, as is the custom. Rabi lives about 21 kilometres away in another village, with her eldest son and his two wives. There are other children in the house, the youngest is aged 5 years.

The house is a traditional walled compound, with individual huts built of clay. The floors and walls are not cemented nor painted, the roofs are mainly thatch, although the newer hut had been recently roofed with corrugated metal sheets. There are few comforts in the compound; minimal furniture - two beds, a table and an armless chair; there is no well or pipe in the house - the village has one borehole and there is no electricity.

Aiye was well cared for by her grandmother who fed her with fried bean cake (*Kosai*) and *pap* or *fura*, a drink made from milled grain balls which have been boiled and blended with sour milk, *maasa* (milled grain dough fried as cake in oil) and an evening meal of *tuo* another milled grain meal boiled and rolled into a thick paste and soup.

Aiye and her grandmother were fond of each other. Rabi carried her about everywhere until recently, when she developed a bad cough, was constantly breathless and too weak to care for Aiye.

A neighbour suggested that Rabi be taken to hospital in Sokoto town. After examinations, the tests showed she had tuberculosis and she was immediately admitted and put on treatment. Meanwhile, Aiye was taken care of by one of the wives in the house but over the course of about three months, Aiye became sickly and on examination it was found that she, too, had become infected with tuberculosis and had to be hospitalized.

Case no. 3

Nana is a thirteen year old girl. She comes from a monogamous family; both parents are educated. Her father is a college teacher while her mother is a caterer. She herself, is attending Junior Secondary School not far from her house in Sokoto. She lives with her parents and two sisters in a well-ventilated, modern house with electricity, running water and a clean environment. Having been born in a hospital, Nana received all her immunizations at the appropriate time and had, until she got the measles, never been infected by any of the childhood diseases for which immunization was available. Her school is about a kilometre away from her house and she usually walks to school. On her way back from school Nana often stops at her mother's friend's house for some time to rest and play with a toddler in the house.

Earlier on, the latter developed measles, Nana came by the house as usual and carried her on a couple of days. It is likely that her infection was from that source.

She was very ill and her mother was very worried but thankfully she recovered, though she lost so much weight and it took some time for her to recover fully.

Case no. 4

Chichi is also a girl aged three and half years. She was born in 1989 in a hospital in Enugu in the south-eastern part of the country by an educated mother who made sure she had all her immunizations. Her father is an administrative officer with one of the Federal Ministries and her mother takes care of her two small children at home.

Chichi lives in rented accommodation in a large compound house with several co-tenants. It is a two-room apartment with shared conveniences. Her father had been transferred to Sokoto from Enugu, and getting a self-contained accommodation was a problem. There were several children in the household and Chichi plays with all of them in the small yard of the house.

During the cold season of 1990, she developed severe measles, like four other children in the compound and was ill for several days. She was admitted to hospital and recovered slowly after treatment.

Her mother could not understand why she got infected especially since she had it on record that Chichi had taken her measles immunization at the appropriate time. For this reason, she had been slow in recognising that Chichi may have had an infection other than malaria for which she was treated at the onset of the fever. It was three days later when her father suggested that his wife should take the child to the hospital where measles was then diagnosed.

An analysis of the case studies

The rest of this paper is devoted to an examination of the cases from the point of view of the medical problems or needs versus the socio-cultural imperative; suggesting possible guidelines and social actions that can be taken to improve the uptake of immunization.

The medical problems

Three communicable diseases were involved in the case studies - measles, tuberculosis and poliomyelitis. We consider below some of the features of the diseases as manifested from statistical notifications as well as the peculiar circumstances that are implicated in their spread.

In the cases in which measles was involved, the readiness with which the disease was spread from an existing case to our two victims is noticeable. Being a droplet infection spread by a virus, both Chichi and Nana came into direct contact with an existing case and it was only a matter of time before they became infected. As Nana is thirteen years, she could hardly be expected to get infected, since the disease has been established as a childhood disease affecting mainly those under five years old. An examination of notified cases in 1975 showed 60% being in this age group (Harris 1975). Working with records from a hospital in Benin, south-western Nigeria 98% of the measles cases were under five (Sinha, 1980). Hence Nana's case is unusual, particularly since she had been vaccinated, albeit several years ago. Chichi's case was also disturbing, she is only three years old and had been immunized against the disease. An infection could have been anticipated since some of her playmates had been infected, had it not been for the immunization. Already it is known that measles incidence in Nigeria is high - for example, the morbidity rates recorded in 1990 is 126.1 per 100,000 people (Table 22.1). Mortality rates are also high - in some hospitals measles account for over 20% of all deaths recorded in paediatric units (Alakija, 1983). Even though measles can be considered endemic in Nigeria, it also shows an almost yearly epidemic pattern. In north-western Nigeria, the peak is between March and June. By August the epidemic could have faded and transmission would have dropped; though there is no month where there are no cases. During the remaining nine months, new susceptibles steadily build up until an epidemic erupts again (Fig. 22.3).

In the tuberculosis case, again close contact was easily established by the already infected grandmother and her toddler-grand-daughter. A bacterial infection caused by mycobacterium tuberculosis in man and *m. bovis* in cattle and other animals, it is transmitted by air-borne droplet - nucleus which contains the bacilli from the patient. In the circumstances under which the little girl lived, it was inevitable that she would have become infected. Her grandmother coughed and disposed of the sputum in any available nook or corner; she was excreting the bacterial all along.

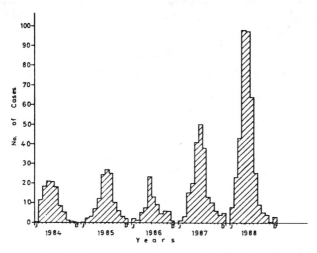

Figure 22.3   Monthly trend of measles admission in Sokoto 1984 - 1988

Table 22.1
Total reported cases and deaths from notified measles in Nigeria 1981-1990

Year	No. of Cases	No. of Deaths	Case Fatality	Case Rates/100000
1981	129,671	1,002	7.72	146.5
1982	139,785	985	7.00	157.9
1983	136,778	983	7.18	154.5
1984	182,591	1,431	7.80	266.3
1985	181,768	1,721	10.60	182.7
1986	115,748	1,991	17.2	130.7
1987	77,566	1,369	17.60	87.6
1988	75,908	968	12.70	85.7
1989	30,436	309	10.10	34.3
1990	111,686	N/A	-	126.1

Source: Federal Ministry of Health Nigeria. Notifiable diseases 1981-90. 1991 official population used as standard.

Tuberculosis has been studied in its epidemiological, pathological and even statistical features in Nigeria (Afonja, 1977; Oriame and Akenzua, 1984; Alakija, 1983). From recent statistical returns of notifiable diseases in Nigeria from 1980-90, - a total of 114016 cases were recorded, with 3,085 deaths and an average case fatality rate of 24.50 per 1000 cases (See Table 22.2).

Table 22.2
Total reported cases and deaths from notifiable tuberculosis in Nigeria 1981-90

Year	No of cases	Cases rates per 100,000	No. of deaths	Cases fatality
1981	10,838	12.24	169	15.57
1982	10,349	11.69	334	32.70
1983	10,212	11.53	208	19.48
1984	10,677	12.06	161	10.78
1985	14,934	16.80	354	25.15
1986	14,071	15.89	515	36.60
1987	13,723	15.50	422	30.75
1988	16,980	19.18	423	24.97
1989	12,232	13.82	300	24.52
1990	20,122	22.90	-	-

Source: Federal Ministry of Health Nigeria, Notifiable Disease 1981-90. Use is made of standard value - 1991 population census.

Again there appears to be a peak period during the cold months of the year January to March; and there are spatial variations also, the northern parts of the country tend to have more cases than the south, a situation which has been attributed to the consumption of unpasteurised milk. (Udomah *et al* 1989). The case of Farouk who suffered from poliomyelitis shows the extent of lack of awareness of the disease which is caused by the polio virus from an infected case. In this instance, it is possible that the child must have got in contact with a carrier or case possible at the crowded Koranic School. It is also known that where sanisation is poor, the faecal - oral route is an important means of transmission. It could be another likely source of infection with paralytic poliomyelitis for Farouk. As it happens both acute and paralytic polio are transmissible in the local environment. Unlike tuberculosis and measles, its prevalence is limited. Between 1981 and 1984 only 133 cases and 2 deaths were recorded in Sokoto State, (Table 22.3).

Table 22.3
Some reported communicable diseases in Sokoto State

Disease	1981 Cases	1981 Death	1982 Cases	1982 Death	1983 Cases	1983 Death	1984 Cases	1984 Death
Measles	12,148	68	5,992	90	10,609	584	22,731	16
Whooping cough	7,758	-	6,565	16	6,807	11	9,213	1
Poliomyelitis	67	2	46	-	18	-	-	-
Tuberculosis	1,287	23	480	6	1,299	18	1,794	9

Source: University Teaching Hospital, Sokoto

The state of immunization as a target for the control diseases

It was in the light of the high prevalence of communicable diseases that immunization has been selected as a possible target intervention for the control of communicable disease. Immunization fundamentally protects the individual with an underlying expectation that a collective group of people could be protected to provide a 'herd immunity'. Prior to 1977, immunization in Nigeria has been limited and it is given to those who voluntarily turn up at "well-baby clinics". Following Alma Ata, the Government decided to embark on an Expanded Programme on Immunization (EPI) which will take that message to all areas and encourage parents to get their children immunized. After undertaking pilot projects, all states worked out the best means of implementing this. By 1980, the expanded programme was well under way in all states of the country.

In Nigeria the extent to which this intervention is fulfilling its objective is yet to be assessed. The cases under study may give clues as to how this intervention is working.

In the cases of Nana and Chichi who both developed measles, immunization has been given in accordance with the laid down schedules. Nana's vaccination was amongst the earlier set of the EPI program towards the end of 1979. She has never suffered from measles until now, twelve years later. A question that needs an answer here is whether she has lost the immunity with the passing years? If so, what would be the immunization of children in that age group who received vaccination at that time - 1979 could there be a need for revaccination? At present there is no such policy and the danger there is that many families who complied with the call for immunization in the early days of the EPI campaign may not be sufficiently vigilant about the possibility of their children becoming infected and may delay to take care.

In the case of Chichi who received the vaccination from age nine months, it can only be surmised that the vaccine was not viable. Indeed, she has not been the only victim. Many children have suffered from measles in spite of the vaccination. Obviously the vaccines may have been unviable at the time of the vaccination.

The case of the paralytic poliomyelitis shows an incompleteness of schedule. He only had one dose of DPT and polio at age four months. His mother did not sufficiently understand the importance of the vaccinations; she was not able to follow up the visits to complete the course. Indeed at the time of the infection, if he had completed the schedule, he would have been due for a booster dose.

The last case of Aiye, who contracted tuberculosis from the grandmother, shows complete lack of awareness of what EPI[2] was all about.

The above cases show a failure of immunization, within these specific contents, to achieve the objectives of protecting the individual against communicable diseases. The underlying causes, as indicated range from peoples' lack of awareness or insufficient appreciation of the programme to vaccine unviability or the disappearance of immunity after a certain period. Clearly the persistence of communicable disease in the developing world can be attributed to both socio-cultural factors and what can be regarded as the system's structural constraints.

In the following and final section we highlight some of the social cultural antecedents and the structural constraints which beset the health care system and require direct addressing if a headway is to be made in disease control.

Socio-cultural bottlenecks and structural constraints

From the cases under study, we notice that the socio-cultural factors which predispose to disease spread cover poor living conditions, substandard housing, inadequate hygiene standards and material deprivation in general. The urban areas display housing shortages which lead to overcrowding.

The state of rural housing is substandard - bare earth floors which make it easy for micro-organisms to survive; windowless rooms which keep stale air unsanitized, and lack of adequate water supply and sanitary arrangements for whole villages. Coupled with the above is the low level of awareness about the causes of illness and the role of personal hygiene and responsibility in ensuring a disease free environment.

All these factors are implicated in the four cases selected for study. The ease with which tuberculosis was transmitted from grandmother to grandchild depicts the palpable material deprivation of many rural families. Even if the child has been immunized, which she was not, it is possible that the infective dose of bacilli would have been high enough to cause tuberculosis. This is in addition to the fact tuberculosis remains an insidious disease with no outward deformities so it goes unnoticed and untreated; making the unrestrained excretion of the bacilli possible. These findings are in line with the radical thinking of earlier contributions to the control of immunicable diseases - (Koch quoted in Dubos 1982). Urban overcrowding is obviously implicated in the spread of childhood infections and the measles case of Chichi is illustrative of this.

Inadequacy of evaluative measures has also resulted in the lack of a revaccination policy which will take care of cases like Nana.

In many ways, medical science in some developing countries has run far ahead of the population. There has been gross inadequacy of effort to improve peoples' knowledge about causation of disease and their role in fomenting the conditions which give rise to those diseases. In other words, health education of basic hygienic practices has been denied to those who have not had the benefit of modern education.

The lack of awareness and ignorance largely contribute to the disinterest shown in immunization and the failure to complete the schedules as is the poliomyelitis case. Merely putting an important preventive service in place without an ancillary machinery for information to all the people, who are to be the beneficiaries, can only mean limited success at controlling preventable diseases. People must be able to have a dialogue with health care providers and have their questions answered and fears allayed. In planning a preventive package which will deal with communicable diseases it is imperative that these sub-groups be recognised and specific approaches be designed to cater for their needs.

A single universal approach for all the social sub-groups as it exists at present is inadequate. People have differential access to information, health messages and even to the care itself; differential responses are also made to calls for participation in the programme. Thus in order to reduce non-challance and non-compliance it would be more appropriate and fruitful to allow the community members in the local government areas to work along with the health care providers.

Furthermore, structural constraints which beset the immunization programme set severe limits on the performance and the level of success at achieving herd immunity. Focusing on the process of immunization is not enough. It is necessary to put into place a comprehensive package that would ensure a smooth running and effective immunization programme. This would require a community that is adequately mobilized to take interest in and contribute to the running of the programme. Such a community could provide assistance when a vehicle transporting vaccines breakdown: they would be able to estimate how long a cold chain has broken down and demand fresh vaccines; they could help remunerate health workers in order to boost their morale. It is only through this that universal coverage can be maintained.

Another requirement is for a concerted national effort to produce the vaccines locally, especially the heat resistant variety. Many rural people have equated immunization with birth control; some do not see the need to 'make' a child sick by vaccinating him when he is healthy; many still remain simplistic and fatalistic in their attitude.

Apart from the socio-cultural hindrances, there are the important structural coordinates which are often lacking and which prevent immunization from achieving its objective of preventing communicable diseases. A discussion with providers indicated that they were often faced with problems beyond their control. The cold chain cannot always be maintained because of frequent disruptions in electricity supply. Sometimes for five continuous days there may be no electricity; vaccines could be rendered unviable in this way. In some areas, vaccines are sometimes not available when they are needed; the supply is not always regular. Breakdown in transportation is another problem which frequently occurs.

Conclusion

The case study approach is germane in bringing to light details of the socio-cultural forces which underpin health care and communicable disease spread in the community. This approach helps to give dues to activities and interventions that must be undertaken if diseases in the community are to be brought under control. In other words, there are unexpected, socially embedded circumstances which cannot be adequately taken care of by adopting a purely biomedical approach to the control of communicable diseases.

The cases discussed show a diversity of social circumstances and the existence of different sub-groups within the local area. Together the programme managers and members of the community can attempt an assessment or evaluation of the interventions set in place for the control of communicable diseases.

Notes:

1. *Matar Auren Kulle* - married women with restricted movement. She lives in purdah or seclusion, except if permission is expressly granted for her to go out during the day time.
2. The EPI programme has a health education unit but they enlighten people who attend the health centres mainly.

References

Afonja, A.O. (1977). 'Observations in tuberculosis and non-tuberculosis patients', *Nig. Med. Pract.* p. 189.

Alakija, W. (1980). 'Immunization of Children in Rural Areas of Bendel State, Nigeria'. *Public Health*, 94.

Alakija, W. (1983). A study of cases of tuberculosis in Bendel State, Nigeria 1975-78 *Nigeria Med. Pract.* 5, 95-8.

Bum, D. *et al* (1986). An assessment of the expanded programmes on immunization in Nigeria. UNICEF Evaluation Publication No. 1.

Chiwuzie, J.C. (1986). 'Immunization in Nigeria, public awareness is inadequate' *World Health Forum* Vol. 7.

Erinosho, O.A. (1989). Health Care and Health Care Service in Nigeria.

Harris, S.C. (1975). Measles in the tropics. *Brit. Journal of Preventive and Social Medicine* 3, 693.

Hopkins, D.R. (1982). The case for Global Measles Eradication. *The Lancet.* June 19.

Oriame O., and Akenzua, G.I. (1984). Contact tracing programme of tuberculosis in Benin City 1981-82. *Nigeria Journal of Paediatrics* II (3), 81-85.

Nigerian Medical Practitioner Journal 1983, 5, (5).

Sinha, N.P. (1980). 'Measles in children under 6 months of age. An Epidemiological study'. *Journal of Hospital Medicine and Hygiene* 83, pp. 255-257.

Udomah, M.G., Edafiogho, I.O. Ware, H.L., Kapu, M.M. and Muhammed, B.Y. (1989). Prevalence of Tuberculosis in Nigeria (1974-83) unpublished mimeograph.

23 Promoting rational drug use in developing countries

Richard O. Laing

Summary

There have been improvements in selection, procurement, distribution, and financing of pharmaceuticals in developing countries over the last decade. This has been primarily due to the Essential Drugs Programme.

The rational use of drugs in such countries, however, remains a problem. A common pattern of polypharmacy, often with brand name drugs or combinations; excessive use of injections and antibiotics; and inadequate examination and dispensing exists in many countries.

To address this issue, indicators of drug use have been developed. Strategies to improve this situation include educational, regulatory, and managerial approaches. To promote rational drug use an International Network for the Rational Use of Drugs (INRUD) has been established.

Introduction

In recent years the WHO Action Programme on Essential Drugs has succeeded in establishing and promoting pharmaceuticals policies in developing countries. The objective of these policies has been to ensure that Essential Drugs (ED) are available to those that require them.

The first element of an essential drug programme has been to select a limited list of drugs to be termed "essential." Over 100 countries now have essential drug list modelled on the WHO Essential Drug Lists (WHO, 1990). Procurement methods have improved such that the price of generic essential drugs has now stabilized or fallen in real terms. Countries still face difficulties in purchasing these drugs due to foreign exchange constraints. Reference price lists are now available.

The distribution of drugs in poor countries with difficult logistic conditions remains a problem. In some countries kit systems (based on military logistics) have been used. In other countries computerized inventory control systems, combined with small district stores and careful transport management, have ensured drug availability.

Considerable attention has been given to the financial management of drugs through revolving drug funds such as the cash and carry system in place in Ghana.

All these developments have improved the availability of drugs, but the problem of how the drugs are used remains.

Drug use in developing countries

The pattern of drug use has been reported from many countries. (Greenhalgh, 1987; Angunawela and Tomson, 1988; Sekhar *et al.* 1981; Hardon, 1987; Hogerzeil, 1988 and Rashid *et al.* 1986). The best systematic study was from Indonesia: "Where does the tetracycline go?" (*Management Sciences for Health, 1988) This study showed a common pattern of polypharmacy, without variation according to diagnosis.*

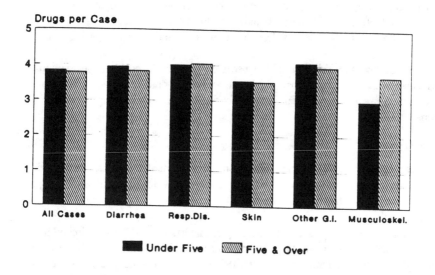

Figure 23.1   Drugs per case by diagnosis. E. Java and W. Kalimantan, Indonesia, 1987

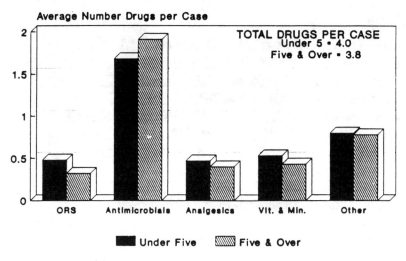

Includes only 'acute diarrhea'

Figure 23.2   Diarrhea treatment pattern, E. Java and W. Kalimnatan, Indonesia, 1987

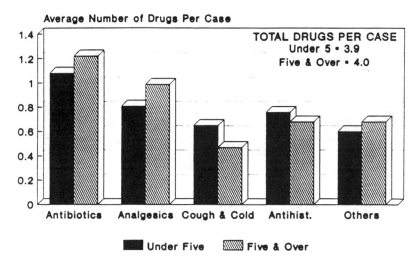

Includes only 'upper resp. infect.' (ISPA)

Figure 23.3   Uri treatment pattern, E. Java and W. Kalimantan, Indonesia, 1987

273

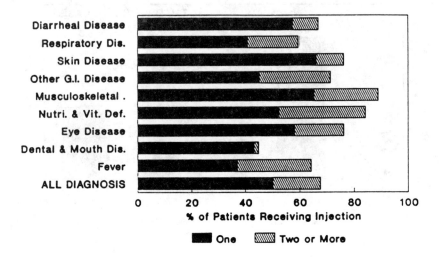

Figure 23.4 **Injection use by diagnosis, E. Java and W. Kalimantan, Indonesia, 1987.**

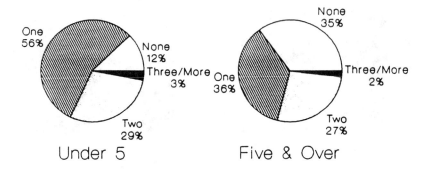

Figure 23.5 **Percent patients receiving antibiotics, E. Java and W. Kalimantan, Indonesia, 1987**

While the depicted data in Figures 23.5 above come from a specific country (Indonesia), they could refer to many developing countries.

The International Network for the Rational Use of Drugs (INRUD) was established by Management Sciences for Health and the Drug Policy Group at Harvard Medical School to address this problem of irrational drug use in developing countries.

Drug use in other developing countries

A study from India by Greenhalgh in 1987 described the widespread polypharmacy, use of combination drugs, and excessive antibiotic use. In Sri Lanka, Angunawela *et al.* (1988) documented drug use in institutions. This again showed polypharmacy and excessive antibiotic usage. Sekhar described a similar pattern of drug use in Ethiopia. A detailed study by Hardon in the Philippines documented the widespread misuse of drugs in a community setting where most of the drugs did not come from the formal sector.

Drug use indicators

To establish a common format for measuring drug use patterns INRUD has developed a set of indicators. These cover indicators of prescribing, patient care, local drug system context, drug supply and consumption, and drug marketing and information. At present, there are 12 core indicators and 7 complementary ones. A simple sampling and data collection from health facilities using prospective or retrospective data has been developed. The indicators have been produced in a manual for WHO and are available from INRUD and WHO/DAP, Geneva

The indicators can be used to describe current treatment practices, compare the performance of regions or health facilities, assess the impact of an intervention, or to periodically monitor drug use performance. The indicators have been circulated and commented upon by INRUD members and other researchers with experience in the collection and analysis of drug use data. The indicators have now been tested in five countries and used in an additional six countries. The definition of these indicators was an iterative process involving circulation, comment, field testing, and large-scale use. The indicators selected are:

Core drug use indicators

Prescribing indicators
1. Average number of drugs per encounter
2. Percentage of drugs prescribed by generic name
3. Percentage of encounters with an antibiotic prescribed
4. Percentage of encounters with an injection prescribed
5. Percentage of drugs prescribed from essential drugs list or formulary

Patient care indicators
6. Average consultation time
7. Average dispensing time
8. Percentage of drugs actually dispensed
9. Percentage of drugs adequately labelled
10. Patients' knowledge of correct dosage

Facility indicators
11. Availability of copy of essential drugs list or formulary
12. Availability of key drugs.

The methods for collecting the indicators have been the subject of intensive study. Large data set from Indonesia, Ghana, Malawi, Honduras, Nigeria, and Tanzania have been used in sampling simulations to determine the minimum acceptable sample sizes. As a result of these studies INRUD recommends for descriptive or comparative studies that:

> Thirty prescriptions should be sampled from at least 20 different sites. Such samples can be collected retrospectively or prospectively. For patient care indicators 30 patients should be observed and interviewed. For drug availability 15 drugs to treat 5 common conditions would be identified and their availability in health centre stores determined. Facility - specific data on the availability of drug information is also required.

This sampling method is based on the observation that variations in practice in an individual prescriber over time or between prescribers within a facility tends to be less than the variations in prescribing between facilities.

INRUD has developed a manual for WHO which became available early in 1993, to detail the definitions and methods for collecting the drug use indicators (MSH, 1991). A public domain software program has been developed to facilitate the entry and analysis of such data.

Interventions to promote rational drug use

Interventions to promote rational drug use can be categorized into:
- Regulatory
- Educational
- Managerial

Each type of intervention has been tested in developed countries, often with unexpected or limited effects (Soumerai *et al*, 1989; Soumerai *et al*, 1990).

In developing countries most emphasis is placed on regulatory approaches (e.g., banning loperamide in Pakistan or drug kits in Ethiopia (Lindtjorn, 1987) or educational efforts (e.g. EDP programs in Zimbabwe (Laing, 1990), Kenya, Uganda, and Tanzania). Very few countries have used managerial approaches.

When interventions have been implemented they have rarely been evaluated. A possible reason for this is the lack of agreed drug use indicators which have now been developed by INRUD/WHO.

Drug use software

To assist in the collection of prescription data, analysis, and report generation, a software package, Rx, has been developed and has now been field tested in a number of countries. The program includes a translation module and a capability to add to the drug list and the problem list, and to add facilities according to levels of care. When all the "bugs" have been removed from the program it will be distributed to assist in the collection of prescription data in a standardized format. This will help in cross-country comparisons and in longitudinal studies to assess impact.

Other areas related to drug use

A considerable literature exists concerning patients' attitude to pharmaceuticals (van der Geest and Hardon, 1990). This is not an area INRUD has concentrated upon. However, it is clearly important, and studies in this area need to be encouraged.

Conclusion

Pharmaceuticals cost developing countries 20-45% of their national health budgets. By seriously addressing the problem of irrational drug use significant savings could be made, the quality of care to patients improved, and the confidence of prescribers increased.

Various interventions (particularly managerial) need to be tested to give policy makers options to choose from when addressing this issue.

References

Angunawela, I. and Tomson, G.B. (1988). 'Drug prescribing patterns: a study of four institutions in Sri Lanka'. *Int. J. Clin Pharmacol The Toxicol 26:69-74.*

Greenhalgh, T. (1987). 'Drug prescription and self-medication in India: an exploratory survey' Soc. Sci. Med. 25:307-18.

Hardon, A.P. (1987). 'The use of modern pharmaceuticals in a Filipino village: doctors' prescriptions and self medication'. Soc. Sci. Med 25: 277-92.

Hogerzeil, H.V. (1988). 'The use of essential drugs in rural Ghana'. *Int. J. Health Services* 16:425-39.

Laing, R.O. (1990).'Rational drug use: an unsolved problem'. *Trop. Doct* 20:101-3.

Lindtjorn, B. (1987).'Essential drug list in a rural hospital'. *Trop. Doct* 17:151-5.

Management Sciences for Health, in collaboration with Yayasan Indonesia Sejahtera and Ministry of Health/Indonesia. 'Where Does the Tetracycline Go? health centre prescribing and child survival in East Java and West Kalimantan, Indonesia'. Jakarta, Indonesia: *Management Sciences for Health*, October (1988).

Rashid, M.U; Chowdhury S.A.R., and Islam N.(1986). 'Pattern of antibiotic use in two teaching hospitals'. *Trop. Doct* 16: 152-4.

Sekhar, C., Raina R., and Pillai K. (1981). 'Some aspects of drug use in Ethiopia'. *Trop Doct* 11:116-18.

Soumerai, S.B., McLaughlin T.J., and Avorn J. (1989). 'Improving drug prescribing in primary care: a critical analysis of the experimental literature'. *Milbank Memorial Fund Q* 67:268-317.

Soumerai, S.B, Ross-Degnan, D., Gortmaker, S., and Avorn, J. (1990). 'Withdrawing payment for non-scientific drug therapy: intended and unexpected effects of a large-scale natural experiment', *JAMA* 263:831-9.

The Use of Essential Drugs. (1990). Fourth Report of the WHO Expert Committee. Technical Report Series No. 796. Geneva: World Health Organization,

Van der Geest, S. and Hardon, A. (1990). 'Self medication in developing countries'. *J. Soc. Admin Pharm* ; 7(4): 199-204.

World Health Organization. (1993). *How to Investigate Drug Use in Health Facilities.* Geneva: World Health Organization,(WHO/DAP/93.1)

24 Drug use in rural and urban Nepal

Kumud K. Kafle, Y. M. S. Pradham, A. D. Shresth,
S. B. Karkee and R. P. Gartoulla

Summary

The average patient attendance per year in the most peripheral health institutions in Nepal is about 13% of the population. About 2.8% of the total population (36.3% of sick population) in rural area is self medicating. Majority of sick population here receive no medication. Self medication is received from different sources, most common being modern drug sellers and Shamans. Large   percentage (78.9%) of self medicating population is not recovered. In the health institutions in rural area, more than 2 items are prescribed in more than 90% prescriptions and more than 40 % of prescriptions have antibacterials. In urban area, more than 24% of prescription has more than two items and antibacterials are prescribed in more than 60% of the prescriptions.

Background

Nepal lies along the southern slopes of the Himalayas. It is sandwiched between India in the South, and the Tibet-region of China in the North. It covers an area of 147,181 square kilometres and runs all along 845 kilometres from East to West and 129 to 241 kilometres from North to South.

Nepal may be divided roughly into four regions namely, Terai, Inner Teria, Hills and Himalayas. Both Teria and Inner Teria occupy 21.4% of the country. Hilly region ranges between 2,700 and 10,000 feet and occupies 44.2% of the total area of the country. Himalaya region lies between 10,000 and 29,000 feet and occupies 34.4 % of the total area of the country.

About 23.3% of the total population (15,022,839) was literate in 1981. 48.7 % of the total literate population had only primary education. About 70% of the total population was in working age group and 65.1% of the total working population was economically active in 1981. Approximately 91.4% of the economically active population was engaged in agriculture and allied activities.

Nepal is a Hindu state and of the total population, 89.5% followed Hinduism in 1981. Buddhists and Muslims comprised 5.3 and 2.7% respectively. Nepal is a multiracial, ethnic, tribal, non-tribal, caste groups and multi-lingual country (Sharma, 1983).

To meet the basic objective of the health for all by the year 2000, the major policies in relation to the implementation of strategies for health for all by the year 2000 are as follows:

1. Basic health services like curative, preventive and promotive will be provided to the rural population through the health posts which are the most peripheral units of the country's health delivery system. These effectively implement Primary Health Care (PHC) activities.

2. In order to increase the effective coverage of population with primary health care services, ward level volunteers programmes will be continued to be implemented in all the 75 districts of the country.

3. The social organizations will be mobilized for primary health care activities so as to avoid duplication of health services and to bring about the effectiveness in the primary health care activities.

4. The Ayurvedic system of medicine will be integrated at the health post and district level.

There was only 96 hospitals, 18 health centres, 816 health posts and 155 Ayurvedic units to serve the population. It is estimated that less than 20% of rural health care is provided by public health care institutions.

Table 24.1
Health institutions and their population coverage (1988).

Estimated population of 1987	No. of hospitals	Hospital population ratio	No of hospitals beds	No of health post	Health post population
17,557,000	96	181,885.42	4,153	816	21,515.93

Each of 75 districts is divided into 9 areas called Ilakas, based on population density and geographic area. Each Ilaka has one Ilaka health post to provide all components of primary health care services. In an 'Ilaka' where there is more than one health post, the rest from the main one will serve as general curative centre (HMG 1991).

Table 24.2 shows average patient attendance in the health facilities in three districts of Nepal (Annual Drug Scheme Report, 1991). There is no consideration on population coverage, morbidity and patient attendance for budget allocation. Supply is quite inadequate and lasts only for few months. There are various drug schemes running to supplement the government supply. But such schemes do not run in all the districts of the country.

Table 24.2
Average patient attendance in the health facilities (1990)

Name of the district	Patient attendance population ratio in hospital	Patient attendance population ratio in health post.
Bhojpur	6%	15%
Taplejung	9%	8%
Panchthar	6%	14%
Average	7%	12.3%

Although there is major difference in patient attendance, annual drug supply is the same for all health posts in all three districts.

In one of the study conducted (Kafle and Gartoulla, 1990) in two village development committees of a district, 3% of the total population (36.0% of the sick population) was found self-medicating (Table 24.3).

Table 24.3
Frequency of self-medication in study villages

Number of households	Total population	Number of sick population	Number of self-medicating population.
319	2050	157	57

Self medication has been defined as any medication obtained without consultation with a qualified allopathic practitioners. It therefore, includes medications obtained in consultation with shamans and other types of traditional practitioners as well as modern drugs sellers.

Majority of the sick population in the study was found untreated.

Self-medication was received from different sources, most common source being modern drug sellers and shamans. (Table 24.4)

When the respondents were asked about their expectation with regard to self-medication more than 80% replied they were hopeful, only 5% had a total belief and 12.3% was using self-medication because there was no other option.

In the health institutions in rural areas, more than 2 items were prescribed in more than 90% of prescriptions (Table 24.5).

Most of prescriptions had antibiotics, as shown in Table 24.6

Polypharmacy and overuse of expensive drugs such as antibiotics is mainly responsible for higher cost of treatment.

On the other hand, study of prescriptions in urban area, 26% of prescription had more than two items and 60% of prescriptions had antibiotics (Kafle et al. 1991; Kafle et al. 1989).

Table 24.4
Sources of self-medication

Sources of medication	Number self-medicating population	%
1. Drug - store	25	43.9
2. Shamans	18	31.6
3. Collecting leaves, grass and herbals.	14	24.6

Table 24.5
Average number of items per prescription (1990).

Name of district	Average number of items per prescription in hospital	Average number of items for prescription in health posts
Bhojpur	2.8	2.5
Taplejung	2.2	2.1
Panchthar	1.7	2.5

Table 24. 6
Average number of prescription containing antibiotics

Name of the district	Average number of prescriptions with antibiotics in hospital.	Average number of prescriptions with antibiotics in in health posts.
Bhojpur	61.9	51.2
Taplejung	41.1	38.2
Panchthar	46.6	56.2

Table 24.7
Number of items per prescription

Number of item	percentageof the prescriptions
1	37.4
2	35.9
3	18.1
4	6.4
5	1.5
6	0.5
7	0.25

Majority of items were prescribed as single drug and single drugs were prescribed mostly under generic name.

Table 24.8
Distribution of prescription items

Prescription item	Generic	Brand	Total
Single drug	223	208	431
Combination drug	15	367	382
Total	238	575	813

Table 24.9
Distribution of antibiotics in out-patient and in-patient departments of a teaching hospital.

Study area	Number of prescriptions studied	Number of prescriptions with antibiotics	%age
Out-patient	404	115	28.4
In-patient	963	639	66.4

There is vast difference in antibiotics prescribing in out-patients and in-patients of the same hospital.

Conclusion

The present chapter discusses drug use in rural and urban Nepal based on different studies. As such there are limited studies conducted in the drug use field.

The paper shows that the majority of the sick population remain untreated. Self-medication is a common practice although most of them do not recover. The paper shows more than two items is a common practice in rural setup than in urban area. This is probably due to lack of or limited diagnostic facilities in the health institutions there. Antibiotics are less frequently prescribed in the health posts than in hospital which has more diagnostic facilities and the prescribers are medical personnel.

Some system of quantifying drugs should be followed and the health institutions should receive drugs accordingly and not on flat basis. This will not only reduce the wastage but also help to bring about more rational use of drugs.

References

Annual Report of The Drug Schemes of The Britain-Nepal Medical Trust - January 1990 to January 1991.

HMG., Ministry of Health (Nepal) and W.H.O. (1988): Country Health Profile.

Kafle, K.K., and Gartoulla, R.P., (1990): A study on Socio-cultural Aspects of Self-medication and its impact on Essential Drug, submitted to WHO.

Kafle, K.K., et. al. (1991) Drug utilisation in out-patient departments in Teaching Hospital. Journal of the Institute of Medicine, March-May.

Kafle, K.K., et. al. (1989) Hospital use of anti-infectives in Nepal, Alliance for the Product Use of Antibiotics, Boston. Newsletter.

Sharma, B.C., (1983) Historical Account of Nepal (In Nepali); Ratna Pustak Bhandar, Katmandu.

25 Awareness and acceptability of the essential drugs list by doctors – a preliminary study in Nigeria

A. F. B. Mabadeje, O. Abosede and A. K. Abiose

Summary

The Essential Drugs Programme (EDP) has been operated in Nigeria since 1986 when the first Essential Drugs List was officially released. Despite the publication of two editions of the National Essential Drugs List (EDL) there has been no published literature on the impact of the EDP on the prescribing pattern of doctors. This study is therefore a baseline against which to judge the effects of the present efforts by the Ministry of Health to spread the gospel of the EDP and to ensure the distribution of the EDL copies to all doctors in the country. The objectives were to document the awareness by doctors of the EDP and the EDL, to see if doctors knew how many editions of the National Essential Drugs List have been printed by the Federal Ministry of Health, to see how many doctors confine themselves to the National Essential Drugs List or Institution List and to find out how the National Essential Drugs List can be improved upon. Doctors from all over the country attending conferences and seminars were individually questioned in line with the above objectives whenever the opportunity arose for encounters with any of the investigators either in Lagos or outside Lagos. Those doctors who were sitting for the postgraduate professional examinations in Medicine or Surgery were also interviewed by one of the investigators.

197 out of 265 (74.3%) surveyed subjects were aware of the EDP. Of the five groups surveyed the Senior Residents were the most aware (89.3%) and the Master of Public Health (MPH) students were the least aware (53.8%). However, only 141 (53.2%) were aware of the National Formulary and EDL. The most aware were the Junior Residents (67.1%) and the least aware were the MPH students. Only 109 (51.1%) had seen a copy of the National EDL, the majority being the Consultants (57.6%) and the fewest being the MPH students (23.1%). Only 78 (29.4%) knew how many printed editions of the National EDL had been produced. The majority were the Junior Residents (37.8%) and the fewest were the MPH students (15.4%). 186 (70.2%) felt that doctors should confine

their prescriptions to the EDL. Majority were the Junior Residents while the fewest were the Consultants. Majority of those who did not wish to confine their prescriptions to the EDL gave the reason that they should be free to prescribe what is best for their patients. Most respondents (92.5%) suggested the free distribution of the EDL to increase its acceptance and majority believed that this goal can best be achieved through the Nigerian Medical Association. The co-operation of doctors must be sought by a programme of education to make them aware of the problem posed by not keeping to an institutional list especially during this period when the subventions to Health institutions by governments are rather meagre and must be parsimoniously spent in order to stretch it to the majority of needy patients.

Introduction

Most of the studies highlighting the prescribing behaviour of doctors as well as drug information to patients have come from the developed countries (Bower & Burkett, 1987; Hull & Marshall, 1987; Nightingale *et al.* 1987; Epstein *et al.* 1984). Publications relating to pharmaco-epidemiology in developing countries have come mainly from Asia and East Africa (Alli, 1988; Ali *et al.* 1986; Aman *et al.* 1986; Angunawela, 1989; Angunawela & Tomson, 1988). Such publications have been few from English speaking West Africa. Mabadeje (1985) in a 1968 study showed that both allopathic and traditional medicine were often combined and that the most frequently used drugs were analgesics and antimalarias. Alubo showed that drugs are marketed and consumed without checks in Nigeria. Abosede in 1984 reported a study of self medication in primary health care in Nigeria. Since then Famuyiwa (1983, 1988), Obaseki *et al* (1987) and Pela (1984) have added to the literature on drug use or issue in Nigeria. Despite the publication of two editions of the National Essential Drugs List (1986, 1989), there has been no published literature on the impact of the Essential Drugs Programme on the prescribing pattern of doctors.

The Essential Drug Programme (EDP) has been operated in Nigeria since 1986 when the first Essential Drugs List was officially released. During medical meetings and symposia as well as during the examination of doctors for the higher professional degrees by one of us (Mabadeje) it has become apparent that a good number of doctors are either still unaware of the essential drugs programme or are reluctant to accept it. Those who are aware of it claim ignorance of the Essential Drugs List. The Federal Minister of Health is keen on spreading the gospel of the EDP to all doctors in Nigeria and determined efforts are now being made to ensure the distribution of the EDL copies to all doctors in the country. This study is therefore a baseline against which to judge the effects of the present efforts by the Ministry.

Objectives

The objectives of the study are to:
- document the awareness by doctors of the Essential Drugs Programme.

- document the awareness by doctors of the Essential Drugs List.
- see if doctors know how many editions of the National Essential Drugs List have been produced by the Federal Ministry of Health.
- see how many doctors confine themselves to the National Essential Drugs List or institution list.
- find out how the National Essential Drugs List can be improved upon.

Methods

Doctors from the different country attending conferences and seminars or sitting for the postgraduate professional examinations in Medicine or Surgery were individually interviewed with questionnaires predesigned in line with the study objectives. The sample was not random but fairly representative as it included doctors at different levels of their profession.

Computer software EPI INFO Version 5 Questionnaire Record was used for data analysis using the following variables: age, sex, professional category (House-Officer, junior and senior residents, postgraduate student in Master of Public Health programme and consultants), Specialty (Medical specialists, Surgical specialities, obstetrics and gynaecology, dentistry) and number of years in practice.

Table 25.1
Number aware of the essential drugs programme

	No surveyed	No positive	%
House officers	109	68	62.4
Junior residents	82	70	85.4
Senior residents	28	25	89.3
MPH students	13	7	53.8
Consultants/CMOs	33	27	81.8
Total	265	197	74.3

Results and discussion

More doctors were aware of the Essential Drugs Programme of the EDL. On the average, more than 50% of all professional categories except Master of Public Health (MPH) students were aware of both. This may be because the MPH students were not actively involved with clinical work at the time of the survey. In a similar study, Angunawela and Tomson (1988) found that only 2 out of 26 (7.7%) physicians at different levels of institu-

Table 25.2
Number aware of the national formulary and essential drugs list.

No surveyed		No positive	%
House officers	109	51	46.8
Junior residents	82	55	67.1
Senior residents	28	13	46.4
MPH students	13	3	23.1
Consultants/CMOs	33	19	57.6
Total	265	14	53.2

-tions in Sri Lanka had heard of WHO Essential Drug List. Our study showed that 53.2% of the doctors interviewed were aware of our national list. It also showed that the most aware group was that of the Junior Residents who were preparing for their residency examinations.

The ignorance of 46.8% is partly due to the communication gap between the staff and heads of institutions or their representatives who attended workshops at which the EDP and EDL were introduced to doctors and pharmacists. It is also partly due to the failure of the Federal Ministry of Health to give necessary financial assistance to the different institutions to enable them to produce their own list and organise workshops to introduce such lists to their staff. That this proportion of doctors is unaware of either the programme or the EDL despite the attempts made by the Federal Ministry of Health to familiarise doctors with the objectives and philosophy of the EDP and the contents of the EDL is an indication of the need for other methods of intensified promotion of the EDL.

Table 25.3
Number who have seen a copy of the national formulary and essential drugs list

	No Surveyed	No Positive	%
House officers	109	34	31.2
Junior residents	82	43	52.4
Senior residents	28	10	35.7
MPH students	13	3	23.1
Consultants	33	19	57.6
Total	265	109	41.1

It is interesting to note that unlike in a previous study (Mabadeje, 1972) where only 6.7% of the doctors interviewed claimed to have seen a copy of the National Formulary and Essential Drugs List the present study shows that there has been an increase in awareness. However, it is still not good enough. Renewed efforts must be made by the Federal Ministry of Health and Human Services not only to produce enough copies of the EDL to go round all doctors and prescribers but to ensure maximum distribution coverage. One of the MPH students remarked that there were copies of the EDL lying in one of the offices of a State Ministry of Health without any attempt to distribute them to would be users. Also, some of those interviewed still believed that the EDP is only for Primary Health Care facilities. A programme to popularise the EDP should therefore be embarked upon by the ministries as soon as possible.

Table 25. 4
Number who know how many printed editions of the national essential drugs list.

	No surveyed	No positive	%
House officers	109	25	22.9
Junior residents	82	31	37.8
Senior residents	28	8	28.6
MPH students	13	2	15.4
Consultants/CMOs	33	12	36.4
Total	265	78	29.4

Table 25.5
Should doctors confine their prescriptions to the essential drugs list?

	No surveyed	No positive	%
House officers	109	84	77.1
Junior residents	82	67	81.7
Senior residents	28	20	71.4
MPH students	13	5	38.5
Consultants/CMOs	33	10	30.3
Total	265	186	70.2

The resistance of doctors to change their prescription habits even in establishments where lists had been produced and workshops held is a cause for concern. Consultants who have prescribed longest and who are used to their old style of prescription were the most resistant even though the preference for freedom to prescribe (Table 25.6) cuts across the different categories of doctors. No doubt, the cooperation of doctors must be sought possibly through an awareness programme to make them recognise the problem posed by not keeping to an institutional list especially during this period when subventions to Health institutions by governments are rather meagre and must be judiciously spent in order to reach needy patients equitably.

Table 25.6
Reason being freedom to prescribe what is best for the patients

	No surveyed	No positive	%
House officers	25	20	80.0
Junior residents	15	11	73.3
Senior residents	8	7	87.5
MPH students	8	5	62.5
Consultants	23	20	87.0
Total	79	63	79.7

Many patients, especially those on treatment for chronic disorders often prefer certain brands of drugs not necessarily because they are more effective, but because of preferable presentation. Sometimes it is because a particular favourite doctor had recommended those drugs in the past. The sentiments of the doctors about having freedom to prescribe what is best for the patient may be closely related to these reasons and is therefore not unexpected.

Table 25.7
How can EDL acceptance be improved upon?

Suggestions	No	%
1. Free distribution of copies to all doctors	245	92.5
2. Distribution by NMA	213	80.4
3. Distribution by NMC	187	70.6
4. Distribution by work place	100	37.7
5. Workshops involving doctors	159	60.0
6. Radio/TV announcements	151	57.0
7. Newspaper advert	125	47.2
8. Newsletters to doctors	102	38.5
9. Involvement of more doctors in production	143	54.0

Appropriate distribution channels must be identified in order to reach all relevant health professionals as soon as possible. Even though the mass media were not highly rated as alternatives for improvement of acceptance they will certainly enhance awareness.

A high proportion of all categories (92.5%, Table 25.7) wanted free distribution of copies of the EDL. Distribution by the Nigerian Medical Association should be explored, being the most favoured channel in this study. However, acceptance and utilisation may not be achieved even if copies are given freely if concerted efforts are not made to promote attitudinal change

References

Abosede, O.A., (1984). 'Self-medication: an important aspect of primary health care'. *Soc Sci Med* 19, 699,

Ali, H.M. (1988). 'Problems in assessing rationality of drug utilization in less developed countries'. *Acta Med Scand* [Suppl] 721, 27.

Ali, H.M. and *et al*. (1986). 'Sudan's new drug policy proves its worth. World Health Forum 7, 256,

Alubo, S.O. (1985). Drugging the people: pills, profits and underdevelopment in Nigeria. *Studies in Third World Societies* 24, 89.

Aman, G.M., Harsana, W. and Adnyana, T.A.K., *et al*. (1986). The use of antibiotics amongst private practitioners. *Indonesian J. Pharmacol Ther* 3 (2), 69,

Angunawela, I.I., (1989). A study of prescribing in rural Sri Lanka. Ceylon Med J 34, 125.

Angunawela, I.I. and Tomson, G.B., (1987). Physicians perception of their own prescribing. Proc. Kandy Soc. Med. 3: 92-94.

Angunawela, I.I. and Tomson, G.B. (1988). Drug prescribing patterns: a study of four institutions in Sri Lanka. Int J. Clin Pharmacol Ther Toxicol 26, 69.

Bower, A.D. and Burkett, G.L., (1987). Family physicians and generic drugs: A study of recognition, information sources, prescribing attitudes, and practices. J. Fam Pract 24, 612.

Epstein, A.M., Read, J.L. and Winickoff, R., (1984). Physician beliefs, attitudes, and prescribing behaviour for anti-inflammatory drugs. Am. J. Med. 77, 313.

Famuyiwa, O.O., (1988). Psychotropic polypharmacy in Nigeria: the danger can be avoided and cost reduced. Trop Doct 18, 7

Famuyiwa, O.O., (1983). Psychotropic drug prescription in Nigeria. Acta Psychiatr. Scand 68, 73.

Hull, F.M. and Marshall, T., (1987). Sources of Information About New Drugs and attitudes toward drug prescribing: an international study of differences between primary care physicians. Fam Pract 4, 123.

Mabaadeje, A.F.B., (1972). The Epidemiology of Drug Usage in Lagos, Nigeria. Proceedings of The East African Medical Society Meeting held in Nairobi pp 221-228.

Mabadeje, A.F.B., Akintonwa, A., Ashorobi, R.B. The value of and effects of implementing an Essential Drugs List in the Lagos University Teaching Hospital. Clin. Pharmacol Ther. 50, 121-124.

National Drug Formulary and Essential Drugs List Federal Government of Nigeria Press. 1986.

Nigeria Essential Drugs List, First Revision 1989

Nightingale, S. and Morrison, J.C., (1987). Generic drugs and the prescribing physician. JAMA 258, 1200.

Obaseki, E.E.E., Akerele, J.O., and Ebea, P.O., (1987). A survey of antibiotic outpatient prescribing and antibiotic self-medication. J Antimicrob Chemother 20, 759.

Pela, O.A., (1984). Psychosocial aspects of drug dependence: the Nigerian experience. Adolescence 19, 971.

Index